THE KARATE-KA

THE KARATE-KA

A SEARCH FOR THE OLD TO UNDERSTAND THE NEW

JOEL REEVES

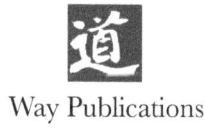

Way Publications

Disclaimer

Please note the publisher and author of this book are NOT RESPONSIBLE for any injury that may result from practising the techniques and/or following the instructions given. Since the physical activities described herein may be too strenuous in nature for some readers to engage in safely, *it is essential that a physician be consulted prior to training.*

Published by Way Publications UK

Copyright © 2015 Joel Reeves
All rights reserved

No part of this publication may be reproduced or utilised in any form or by any means, electronic or mechanical, including photocopying, recording, or by any information storage and retrieval system, without prior written permission from the author.

Author website:
www.thekarateka.com

ISBN: 978-0-9559876-2-5

First Edition 2015

To
Isyado Hirokazu
伊舎堂博和

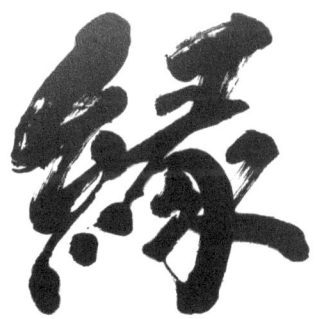

Destiny.
Fate meant for this to happen
- This must have happened for a reason.
                                    HIGA YUGEN

ACKNOWLEDGEMENTS

In addition to the generosity of teachers and friends who have guided and shaped me along the Way, this work ultimately reached fruition due to the early encouragement, support and assistance of the following people:

THE KOMORIYA FAMILY, ATSUMI IKEMIYAGI,
TOMOKO ITOKAZU, EWAN A STEWART,
MARK LITHGOW, PAUL VERMEHREN,
DONOVAN HARRY & COLLEEN WATSON

SPECIAL THANKS TO

MAGDALENA, for your tireless support and sustained words of encouragement
"Just finish the book already!"

Contents

1. A rude awakening   1
2. Check your watch   8
3. Big trouble in little Tokyo   17
4. Furosha   22
5. Lost and found   35
6. Knock knock   42
7. Finding balance   52
8. The Old Man in the park   62
9. Whispers from the past   73
10. Te Time   83
11. Letting go   94
12. Goodbye   104
13. Okinawa   115
14. Sipping Te   126
15. Koza   135
16. Kaminchu   147
17. A dog named Shen   158
18. FM21   167
19. Change   178

EPILOGUE: The old, the new   188

1
A rude awakening
"Shotokan punches don't work"

Tokyo. 1994. I'm eighteen years old, standing in my underwear wiping the sleep from my eyes. The teacher, still drunk from the night before, is patting his belly and goading me in front of the others. "Hit me!" I glance around the dojo that is our makeshift dormitory. Shell-shocked and exhausted I'm not entirely sure I've had any sleep since arriving from London a few days ago. "Come on! Hit me! - Make a stance. Reverse punch!"

It's futile. Anyone who has practiced karate for any length of time knows that the muscles of the stomach can be trained to such a degree as to take the hardest of punches. It proves nothing. But there's another reason why I don't want to participate. I know that this will become yet another demonstration to the rest of the group that the karate style I learn, Shotokan, is inferior to the style they learn. This game has been going on since we arrived. Was it two days ago or three? I'm really not sure.

"Come on. Do it. Punch!" I can't see a way out of it. Reluctantly I adopt *zenkutsu-dachi*, the 'front stance' of karate and take aim. But I've already lost. If I manage to strike hard enough to knock him down I feel that either a) he'll get up and kill me or b) the others will kill me before I can run out onto the street. And yes, the intensity of the moment feels that bad.

Drawing a deep breath I concentrate upon his belly and clench my fist. My audience consists of about sixteen guys, the youngest of which is almost ten years my senior. Since we left England all but three of them have been doing their best to keep me on edge. They throw feint punches as I pass them, try to isolate and intimidate me or generally act hostile. It's like being on a school trip and finding yourself the odd one out in a class of delinquents. The teacher is either never around at the right moment, or worst, acting as threatening as they are. At other times it seems like everyone is playing the 'good cop, bad cop' routine - except every few hours they all change roles so you really don't know who to trust.

THWACK! Driving my right fist forward it corkscrews through the air as my left hand simultaneously clenches and draws back close to the hip. With perfect form the punch lands hard, my wrist doesn't buckle. But the moment I do this a cupped palm slaps heavy upon the crown of my head sending a searing pain that pierces my core and causes white stars to sparkle in my eyes.

"No! Punch harder!"

I growl and try to shake off the stinging pain. Scuffing the ruffled bedding away from under my feet I take a stronger stance. Through blurred eyes I see my audience watching in awe of their teacher. This time I concentrate the force of the strike to penetrate deeper, to travel through its target. I'm tempted to land the punch in his solar-plexus, perhaps it would have more effect? Self-preservation advises me against it.

'EEYAH!' I drive it home with a low *kiai*, a karate 'power shout'. Twisting my hips fully into the strike and snapping the fist back out just as fast. Again his palm slaps hard upon my head. My legs buckle. I back off. Pain and humiliation. With a clenched jaw and teary eyes I shoot daggers across the room. My heart is pounding and my senses are screaming at me to get away. Whenever I'm around this group it's like there's an oppressive vibe bathing the room keeping me on high alert. Not for the first time I consider taking the *wakizashi* short sword off the wall behind me and going down in a berserk fury.

The teacher shakes his head with contempt and waves his hand as if to dismiss me. He turns to the group and begins, as expected, a sermon about the ineffectiveness of Shotokan punches.

I retreat to the shower. I think about how I'm going to get away from this crazy lot while I still can. I also think about why the Shotokan punch doesn't work…

*

Shigeru Egami, was a senior student of Gichin Funakoshi, the man largely responsible for introducing karate to the mainland of Japan from its native Okinawa during the 1920s. Like me Egami also experienced disappointment in the Shotokan punch. He once wrote:

'Among the problems I studied, and sometimes had to study over again, was how to avoid injury to the wrists, elbows and shoulders. The first realization that lead to a solution was that the human body, being a living thing, is very elastic. If power is concentrated in the wrist or the elbow or the shoulder, it will return to the place of concentration. If you spread out your elbows or raise your shoulder, power will escape from those places.'

It's not an easy pill to swallow, learning that the punch you've spent years perfecting doesn't work. But the Shotokan punch is ineffective for several reasons. Firstly the point of contact is the two largest knuckles of the index and middle finger with the fist fully overturned from palm side up to palm down at the moment of impact. The weakest point is the wrist itself as through constant compression over years of training the soft tissues are compounded and many advanced karate-ka complain of stiffness and arthritic type aches in the area. If the wrist is not well trained in this position it is likely to buckle when hitting something hard such as a *makiwara* striking post causing more pain to the puncher than their target.

To combat this, karate students often tense the fist and brace the wrist before impact. But this contraction of muscles in the arms and chest actually reduces the outward flow of force into the target. To further guard against injury many students instinctively tense the shoulder muscles to 'brake' the speed of the punch incase it misses the target altogether or, as when training with no target, to prevent damage to the elbow through hyper-extension. This tensing of the muscles coupled with anchoring the feet in a 'power-stance' is what reduces the overall speed and delivery of the blow and disperses physical muscular power in the opposite directions of the target. Tensing the shoulders sends it upwards and tensing the elbow sends it to the side.

There is a secret to improving the effectiveness of the punch though. Relaxed power. Funakoshi would tell students "become not hard but soft". In post war Japan the message was lost. 'What was the old man talking about? We do karate to become hard, not weak.' But at the end of the Second World War Japan was physically and spiritually smashed. A foreign force occupied their land and restrictions were placed on the study of martial arts. America had felt compelled to drop two atomic bombs as a last resort to dealing with an enemy that used suicide as a justified means of warfare.

In a private correspondence, years later, I questioned a senior tutor of the Okinawan Theatre Group as to why he felt there was a shift from learning the softer, more circular, movements of cultural art-forms such as martial arts and dance, with the more robust, staccato movements of today. He surmised that:

'After the war Japanese males generally felt emasculated compared to the occupying US marines. At this point many lost faith in the 'old ways' and instead sought to develop powerful physiques similar to western athletes; so as to feel like valid men in a modern world.'

This period also correlates with a shift in where a martial artist generates power from. Prior to the war everything was *hara* based; all movement coming from the anatomical centre of gravity located a few inches below the navel. Since the war a cruder power generated from shoulder development has become the preference of zealous students, and for those teachers schooled before WWII it has become a constant source of correction for the younger generations. "Drop your shoulders!"

It would take me another decade of training before I was finally instructed 'how' to develop a true *hara*. Such is the rarity of teachers, both Japanese and foreign, who are skilled in its proper application.

Back in 1976 Egami reflected upon watching Funakoshi practicing on the *makiwara*:

'It seemed to me that Master Funakoshi hit the striking post very lightly, uttering words that sounded like "hoi, hoi." At that time, I thought that he was not striking forcefully and attributed it to his being of small stature and already about sixty years of age.'

He goes on to comment on the masters third son Gigo:

'...his blows were terrific. One thing I could not understand: While he told us to strike from the hips, he himself took a stance more like a horse-riding stance and aimed his blows at the striking post from a position with his hands dangling from his sides, without using his hips much. But there was no questioning the power of his blows as he lunged forward with all his body weight behind them. He frequently broke the striking post in two.'

When I teach about relaxed power I think about an old wooden figurine toy that would naturally stand straight but when you pushed a button underneath its base it would go floppy. When this button was released the figurine would again spring back to attention through the aid of elastics. The changing movement of this toy is like the feeling of punching with relaxed power.

So is the Shotokan punch ineffective? Yes and no. As it is practiced in a dojo today the punch is in its basic '*kihon*' form. It is a training device that actually is doing a lot to develop the muscle structure of the arms, shoulders, stomach and waist. In so doing it's also building a protective layer of muscle over several 'vital' targets. When training in Japan one will often witness teachers liberating basic movements from form and applying them in different ways. I recall a session in which a young instructor broke the standard corkscrew punch into three parts. The first was the half-way position, in which the punch became a solid low-level uppercut jab to the ribs or sternum. The next was the regular punch in full range and the third was the draw back of the lead arm as a rear elbow strike. Three techniques being developed through one 'long-form' technique, the corkscrew punch.

Earlier sparring matches with the group I was with had already revealed to me, with a painful awareness, the vulnerability of the Shotokan punch in its full position. At the final moment the top of the wrist is dangerously exposed to a knuckle strike from an opponent employing such short-range tactics, and it's equally at risk to a downward elbow strike from someone's guard.

Years later I would learn that when Funakoshi originally learnt the punch from his teacher Itosu it was actually delivered as a quarter turn and never a full corkscrew. In this way the largest knuckles still struck the target but the fist landed in a diagonal position with the elbow down and top of the hand less exposed to a counter attack.

The incident with group that morning had highlighted and brought to the surface a deep rooted doubt within me about the effectiveness of Shotokan as a combative art. I was under no illusion that the techniques used by them were far more geared towards fighting than mine were. Perhaps that needn't be a problem in itself, but most teachers in a Shotokan dojo will lead their trainees to believe that their punch is overly effective, that one strike is all it takes to knock someone down. And that can lead to a false sense of confidence.

…Rinsing the suds down the drain I paused in the shower and considered my options. Should I stay or should I go? If I stay there might be trouble.

When I opened the small cubicle door I froze for a moment. One of the group who I sensed disliked me the most was waiting in the corridor outside. He scowled and shook his head.

"Pathetic. The next time he stands there like that and says 'hit me' you should punch him in the face as hard as you can."

I blinked. To this day I'm not sure if he genuinely meant it as supportive advice or out of some hope that I would actually follow his words of wisdom and in so doing get far more than a pat on the head.

2
Check your watch
"Our Grandmaster controls both time and space"

Day two. Or is it three? The group is milling about in an excited mood because today they are going to have a special session with the 'Grandmaster'. Some are having breakfast in the kitchen while others are rolling away their futons from the dojo floor.

The owner of the house, himself a very capable master of karate, passes me and beams his warm friendly smile. I've not had much opportunity to speak with him. I understand he is fluent in five languages, English being one of them. He seems the sort of person who can make people feel at ease just by being around. I've since discovered it a quality of many good karate-ka. He wont be going to the 'special session' today as he has reached a stage in his karate where he no longer trains with The Grandmaster and is developing his own way.

Yesterday I was told I would be welcome to stay as a live-in student when the rest of the group leaves Japan in two weeks time. The dojo floor would be my bedroom and in exchange for keeping the place 'tip top' I would receive personal instruction in karate. It's an honour to be offered such an opportunity and one that I've been seriously considering. Except one thing keeps changing my mind. 'The Group'. Right now I doubt I will survive two weeks without something kicking off and me ending up in hospital or the harbour.

I packed my bed away and thought about slipping off to spend the day on my own when the teacher of the group saw me.
"Ah there you are." My shoulders tensed, half expecting another smack on the head. "Listen, I know you don't train in *'our style'* but I really think you should come along today and meet The Grandmaster. He doesn't usually allow outsiders but for you he is prepared to make an exception." I make a face and try to politely back out but he's insistent, and actually he isn't really asking, he's sort of telling me.
"It's a once in a lifetime opportunity for you."
Seeing as I've still not been able to contact the dojo of my choice, and with no other plans, I decide to go. I reason that if after today I don't feel welcome in the group I'll leave.

I'm glad I went. It became one of the most defining moments in my life and significantly altered my view of karate and martial arts from that day on. I will never forget stepping into that dojo, it was like stepping back in time, even the air seemed old. Located down one of countless side streets The Grandmaster's dojo was actually a little home with lots of green plants growing outside. His front room 'was' the dojo and as I remember it now he sat in a sort of alcoved recess with a little dog by his side.
On the whole I've always found the Japanese extremely warm and welcoming. I don't doubt that once you were in his circle this Grandmaster had a big heart too. But first impressions last and although my first impression had undoubtedly been tainted somewhat by my experiences with The Group - "*Our Grandmaster plays with people like Kanazawa*", another throw away comment presumably intended to undermine my interest in Shotokan, I felt he looked upon me now with suspicion. It was like I'd come to steal his secrets, and yet I swear it was him rummaging around in my mind when he looked at me. In either case he was not someone you warm to easily and had, I felt, a murderous air about him. A regular old

man on the surface but one who had the ability to kill you effortlessly in a fight and think nothing of it.

High on one wall there were stacks of old white karate uniforms, rolled and stained yellow with sweat, pushed onto long wooden pegs.
"These were left by students who couldn't hack the training." Someone told me. "They were so scared they ran out the door and left them behind!' He added, with a look of conceit on his face as if to say 'we are tough'. I wondered why, If they were 'that' scared, did the owners wait to change out of their uniforms before running off?' But it seemed this place encouraged those kind of rumours. In one corner sat an old metal gas drum with makeshift rubber arms and worn-out karate belts tied to it. *'Makiwara'* I was told, which wasn't a rumour, it was a crude looking striking post. The whole place was small and cramped for the number of us now filling the floorspace. Then a second group arrived too.
The teacher beckoned me over and spoke in hushed tones.
"Okay, I've spoken with O'sensei and he says you can join in. How much money do you have on you?" At once I felt I'd walked straight into another trap and started to see a pattern forming.
I'd arrived in Japan with an amount of cash to see me through what was effectively a week long festival; 'Golden Week'. As it happens Golden Week was the reason I was stuck with the group in the first place and not training in Shotokan at the headquarter dojo of Hirokazu Kanazawa. 'My dojo' had closed for the festival which only added to the fuel of the taunts that I didn't study a 'real' karate style because 'their dojo' never closed. "It's open all year round twenty-four hours a day." The rest of my funds were in a bank account so I could draw on them later, but for now even the banks were closed and I still had most of the week to go.
In order to get to Japan and follow my dream I'd spent two years since leaving school working four menial jobs a day. The first evening I felt obliged to contribute to a social 'kitty' along with everyone else. A kitty which was meant to last a while but

had already been dwindled by one member spending the first night in a local 'love hotel'. Furthermore the group was only here for two weeks and wanted to party hard. For most of them it really was a once in a lifetime experience. For me it was the start of a new period in my life. I was on a shoe-string budget intending to stay as long as I could. On top of paying for my bedding and staying at the dojo, which I was seriously considering abandoning ten days early. my initial funds were starting to diminish through visits to bars, restaurants and excursions I wasn't really interested in. A request for more money seemed to accompany each one.

"How much does the training today cost?" I asked.

"No. The training today doesn't cost anything but you need to give The Grandmaster a gift. It's customary. We all bought him something from home but you need to make your own gift - hurry up, how much do you have on you?"

Taking out my wallet he took it from my hand and fanned through the notes. Training for the afternoon was to cost me a little over two thirds of my remaining cash. "This is enough. Okay, go sit down."

"*Konichiwa*. Hello." We all huddled close on the floor as an interpreter introduced The Grandmaster and went through the days itinerary. "As you can see. The time on your watch is different to the time on our clock." Next to me a couple of Americans were checking the time and nudging each other with bewildered looks. I didn't understand. Time-zones? Surely the clock is either fast or slow? The interpreter continued in short clipped sentences. "This is because. Our Grandmaster controls both time and space." There were a few gasps and even an "oh gee". I still didn't get it. "It's true" another member of the group leaned in and whispered to me. "He can restart stopped watches, bend spoons and everything." He pointed to his head and mouthed "With his mind."

Party tricks aside I didn't think that was quite what the interpreter was suggesting. Later that day I started to see it more as 'controlling timing and distance' in a combative sort of way. If you can control the distance between yourself and an opponent then you also control, to an extent, what type of attacks they can use to strike you. In simplistic terms, the further away someone is then the longer it will take for them to hit you. If the distance is short then the opposite is true. Real combat can be far more subtle than that. Therefore by controlling space, distance, you control the timing of your opponent's attacks.

On a deeper level the expansion of space creates time and our brain can be influenced and tricked into experiencing the passage of time in different ways. It's called a temporal illusion; a distortion in the perception of time. Have you ever suddenly looked at an analogue clock and felt that the second hand stops moving or even moves backwards 'just' as you looked at it? What about when an alarm-clock wakes you up and you hit snooze - only to fall back asleep and feel like no time has elapsed when it next goes off? Or have you ever woken from a dream in which a sudden external sound or event has actually been playing an observable role in your dream-state? Dream time is slower than our experience of waking time. Through combat this Grandmaster had techniques that enabled him to influence an opponent's perception not only of time but other phenomena as well.

After the introduction we relocated to train at a local high school as there were too many of us to do anything in the Grandmaster's front room. We walked in our *gi* through the side streets of this old part of Tokyo renowned for some of its classical architecture. Neighbours gave us curious, yet knowing, looks. I imagined the Grandmaster was a local hero of sorts. It is said that after the war, when times were hard, fights would sometimes break out in a small square behind the school. When things got really out of hand the neighbours would rush to his house and he'd quickly come to settle things, usually by punching everyone involved and leaving them face down on the ground where they fell.

This tale reminded me a lot of a story Funakoshi recounted about his teacher Itosu:

'...*Itosu was set upon by a group of young thugs, but before long the hoodlums were all lying unconscious in the street. An eyewitness, seeing that*

Itosu was in no danger, rushed off to tell Itosu's friend Azato what had transpired. Interrupting his account, Azato said, "And the ruffians, of course, were all lying unconscious, with their faces to the ground, were they not?" Much surprised, the witness admitted that that was true, but he wondered how Azato could have known. "Very simple," replied the master. "No karate adept would be so cowardly as to attack from the rear. And should someone unfamiliar with karate attack from the front, he would end up flat on his back. But I know Itosu; his punches would knock his assailants down on their faces. I would be quite astonished if any of them survive.'

What kind of punch would cause someone to fall face down? I reasoned it would need to hit like a bullet. It would be fast. Propelled forward with nothing but air behind it and hitting as heavy as lead. It would strike with a whiplash-like effect and probably cause extreme concussion. By shaking the victims brain in their skull. the nervous system could shut-down and then, loosing motor-function, their legs would give way and their head lull forward until they hit the ground. Nowadays, in self-defence, you'd have to be careful of using such a punch just incase your attacker injured themselves as they hit the ground and sued you afterwards. Assuming of course they survived at all.

Back in the high school gymnasium the content of the 'special session' consisted largely of *kata* and *bunkai*. If *kata* are choreographed sequences of karate techniques, performed much like a military parade drill or ritualised ballet, then *bunkai* is the practice of those techniques with a partner for combat and self-defence.

Shotokan had lots of *kata*, twenty-six, but no *bunkai*. This style had half as many *kata* and lots of *bunkai*.

In fact, their whole style was extremely combat focussed. If *kata* is the solo practice of karate techniques, and *bunkai* the practice of those techniques in a semi-pre-arranged fashion with a partner, then *kumite* is using those techniques in any way you like against a partner doing the same back at you. Modern Shotokan has a whole set of '*kumite*' exercises that are mostly pre-arranged in that both attacker and defender know exactly what technique is coming and when. These drills are used to isolate and develop key skills required for a competition styled match; footwork, distancing, timing etc. These guys trained a different way. It had nothing to do with sport.

When they engaged in *kumite* the two fighters faced each other with a distance of about fifteen feet between them. It was slow at first. The fighters closed the range carefully, moving like snakes, then crouching tigers, and then elegantly like regal cranes. The engagement opened like a game of chess, each side tactically advancing in such a way as to limit the opponent's opportunity to attack. And then the clash. A final decisive moment with a clear victor. In Shotokan, fighters rushed in, the head and torso being the only valid targets. But here anything was a target. If your stance was too wide you'd get a kick to the groin. Too long and it was your knee. The risk for serious injury was high and you quickly learnt not to make silly mistakes.

The first day I trained with The Group was a brisk Sunday morning. The air was so cold it almost stung the nostrils when you breathed. Fingers and ears were numb. I witnessed a guy get his nose broken. The cracking sound of fist meeting skull and cartilage ripping lingered in the air and haunted me for a while to come. Another time a student painfully buckled their toes upon my knee as I instinctively covered his kick to my groin; a testament to how hard the kick was intended to land.

Just a week before we left for Japan another trainee broke his shin when someone blocked his kick. He spent the whole trip being wheeled around in a chair or awkwardly managing on crutches. To me he was one of the 'good guys'. He didn't say much to me but he didn't really make me feel on edge either.

In Shotokan we learnt phrases like '*unsoku*' and '*maii*'; footwork and striking distance. This group learnt things like octopus technique, hypnosis, *ki*, rhythm and 'crane technique'. The latter being a way of vibrating the body, either to induce an adrenaline release or perhaps to release the stress of one. Many animals vibrate after surviving a threatening encounter to release tension in the nervous system and disperse unspent adrenalin from the body. Humans have generally lost this ability but here these guys learnt how to bring it on at will.

Despite the intense unwelcoming feeling I got from The Group I was enamoured by their fighting technique. It was all at once raw, real and brutally effective.

Training was also less regulated. In Shotokan I was used to marching up and down the dojo in regimented lines making a terrible racket whilst kicking and punching the thin air. Here, in the large school gymnasium, people worked in pairs and small groups. They shared and discussed experiences and feelings, they helped each other develop. It was a brotherhood. Despite the dent in my finances which, I was assured, had made me a lifelong member to the dojo, and my future children too, The Grandmaster left a lasting impression upon me. He touched me. Quite literally.

At one point in the session he gathered everyone around to demonstrate a painful joint locking technique on my arm. I remember looking down at his feet paralysed with pain. They were pale with liver spots and yellowed calluses from years of kicking things. I was torn between 'tapping out' or not. I thought that if I tried to signal to him he might think I was trying to attack again and so crank the technique some more. Suddenly the grinning face of my Japanese training partner leaned down into view. "If you don't submit he will shatter your elbow." I submitted.

After I dusted myself off I was told,

"If you throw a punch at sensei you are enemy. He will break your arm or kill you. Right now he has sent *ki* to your heart." I rubbed my elbow. It was true. A curious, aching, vibrating feeling was now resonating from my arm and slowly moving into my chest.

"But he told me to attack? It was a demonstration!" I protested. "Doesn't matter." The student laughed. "You still enemy." I laughed too and we continued training.

In the presence of the Grandmaster it did seem that some strange things were happening. When he first saw me it really did feel like he was invading my mind, and there was all that talk about stopping watches and things.

Something else happened that afternoon too. The leader of the second group had been a student of the Grandmaster for a long time but that day he kept asking questions. I assumed he must have been writing a book or something because he didn't stop mining for knowledge. Everyone was getting a bit annoyed. It was annoying. I think The Grandmaster knew we were all getting fed up too. He was going to have to deal with this and I guess he was just waiting, or creating, the right time to do it.

"O'sensei - what is the meaning of a three day death strike?" The hall fell silent. It was one question too many and you didn't need to be a master to sense the group's general thoughts. The enquirer was to become the subject of his own enquiry.

With the help of the interpreter the Grandmaster proceeded to demonstrate the legendary 'delayed death touch' of karate. The movement he used was similar to a double hammer-fist strike that landed almost simultaneously on each side of his opponent's ribs causing him to sink and go ghostly pale.

"Usually." The interpreter began. "The *ki*, would enter one side of the body. Then leave, other side. But. Sensei has sent energy in both sides. The *ki* cannot escape. It just bounce inside. Damaging organs. In three days. Enemy die." He added with a sort of matter-of-fact shrug "Kill or be killed." Some people smirked, but when the Grandmaster then pulled open his 'enemy's' *gi* there was a curious feint red mark growing in the middle of his victims chest. Like ET.

Had I just witnessed the coveted 'Death Touch' of karate? The immediate effect of the strike was that it stopped the incessant questioning. But would it also stop his heart? All I can say is that after that day I never saw the teacher again.

He didn't die though. I never saw him again because of events thats unfolded later that evening which would cause me to leave the group once and for all.

3
Big trouble in little Tokyo
"Kill or be killed"

After the special training session at the Tokyo high school everyone went to a restaurant to celebrate, catch up with old friends and make new ones. The Grandmaster sat at the head table with the other sensei and a few of the foreign students. Judging by the excitement I suspect he was fixing watches and manipulating cutlery. I sat further back with the rest of The Group and avoided getting drunk. I wanted to remain clear headed because I knew the others wouldn't. And that made my situation with them all the more risky.

For example. Last night we came back from the bath-house on the train and everyone was drunk. Especially the teacher. He began teaching a secret technique which in most places would be considered anti-social. Spitting.

"When an enemy faces you, you must do everything to win. It's kill or be killed." He hissed like a snake and pulled a demonic face before forcefully projecting saliva from his mouth and flurried some lightening fast punches in the air. "Distraction! Then attack! Understand? Kill or be killed." His fingers splayed like a cranes wings as he stood rooted in a fighting stance while the train rocked along the tracks. It was uncomfortable viewing and the few Japanese 'salarymen' making their way home late in the night filtered out of the carriage one by one with nervous expressions upon their faces.

When we got back to the dojo no one wanted the night to end so they went out again in search of a local bar. I stayed in with two of the 'good guys' and used the opportunity to get some much needed sleep. I reasoned that if I could be asleep by the time they all got back I'd be relatively 'out of mind' and safe.

As it happened the others came back in staggered pairs throughout the early hours of the morning. I tried not to stir, willing myself to remain concealed in shadow; trying to become 'one' within the ruffled shape of my bedding. I drifted in and out of an uneasy sleep while their quiet murmuring voices spoke of karate, their trip, me. And other things I found curious.

"He's looking for a real dojo. But he doesn't know he's already found it."... "Shotokan is weak."... "Academy style karate." ... "How can he not want to learn a real Way?"... "Our way."... Were they trying to brainwash me? At other times they spoke of their teacher. They placed him high upon a pedestal.

"When my father dies 'he' will become my father."

"Yes. 'He's' more like a father to me than mine ever was."

I wondered what would make men in their late twenties and early thirties speak that way. My upbringing was reasonably stable and my brothers and I were all encouraged to be independent from an early age. By fourteen I had a converted studio away from the main house. At sixteen I tried to join the army but failed a medical exam. I bounced back and set my sights on Japan. Now, at eighteen, I was here but I'd never felt the need to seek a 'father figure'. I guess I already had one and was ready to make my own way without his guidance. Surely that's a natural phase to reach?

CRASH! The door to the dojo burst open and I sat up just in time to see a demon come bundling in, tripping over sleeping bodies and rolling forward to his feet "I want to fight someone!" He looked possessed. "Come on! Lets go out - we'll find someone and…" The others hurriedly hushed him up. A few grumbled from their sleep and a couple tried to appease him, they reasoned it was late and none of them felt like drinking anymore. Also our host and his family were asleep upstairs. so someone put the kettle on and the commotion eventually died down. Perhaps it was a bad dream? I drifted back into a troubled sleep unaware that in a couple of hours time I'd be demonstrating my punch to a hungover and easily impressed audience.

After the restaurant we said goodnight to The Grandmaster and headed for a bar. It was mild outside. A light drizzle hung in the air causing the flashing neon lights above us to glisten on the tarmac streets below. Taxis and cars inched along in short stop, start motions. Pachinko parlours rattled and chimed as players caused thousands of little silver balls to tumble through the amusement machines. Down side streets pretty hostess girls called out in broken English trying to tempt us into their establishments. Some of them wore traditional kimonos and wooden clogs whilst sheltering from the rain beneath clear plastic umbrellas with 'hello kitty' printed on them. Others wore less.

The bar we chose was above street level. I have no idea where. It was cramped and we occupied several tables that soon collected an array of empty glasses. I sat on a bench seat sandwiched between two members of the group. That's when he came up to me.

I'd only met him once before. He was a giant. Towering above me he placed a large heavy hand upon my shoulder, sniffed the air and swayed drunkly. His dark voice slurred as he raised a fist.

"Don't move." He had the look and build of a world-class heavyweight boxer. I half felt he was one, but I couldn't place his name. Just one of his fists was bigger and meatier than both of mine put together. This was new territory and it was dangerous.

If I had to place everyone in the group on a scale of hostile to pleasant he would have been quite far from hostile before this moment. Whereas a fair few had been trying to make me flinch with fake punches and quick sneers throughout the trip this guy never had. He seemed, reasonable. Quiet. A gentle-giant. Now he seemed drunk, unpredictable and threatening. For all I knew he might just be having a bit of fun at my expense, but like Lennie and his puppy in the story 'Of mice and men' his innocent enough actions could end up having a detrimental effect upon my wellbeing. I couldn't take that chance.

Then something happened I'd never experienced before. In my mind everything went calm, thoughts quietened. The din of the bar became faded and muffled, like standing outside a nightclub. The world around me fell away. It was just him and me. Time itself seemed to slow and a definite thought formed. 'I wont flinch. If his fist passes a certain point I will react.' And that's exactly what happened.

He swung his heavy punch towards the side of my head and in the blink of an eye I shot from my seat into his opening and thrust my hand straight to his throat. His eyes rolled upwards and he collapsed in a heap on the floor like a sack of potatoes.

I was stunned. Looking at my hand, shaped as it was in a Y, the thumb had struck a point on the side of his neck where the pulse throbs heavy. 'Where had that technique come from?' My mind scanned through the twenty-six *kata* I knew and I couldn't place it. It was an instinctive response. Effortless. Untrained but perfectly timed.

At once everything started to rush back in. The sounds of the bar and the people around me. My calm mind shattered by confusion. I glanced to the exit. Someone touched my arm, a 'good guy'. The teacher glared over from his table, he looked angry and embarrassed in front of the Japanese group.

"What's going on?" He demanded. I tried to protest my innocence but I was already in the wrong.

"Get him out of here! You're scaring the locals!" Two good guys said they'd go back with me and we hurriedly left the bar.

Of course you read about the effect of pressure-points and hear stories, but until that moment I had never felt it or even fully believed what I read and heard. The opponent was easily twice my size and he fell so quickly, like I'd just switched him off. By all accounts it was a strange and scary evening but something had awoken in me.

Response without conscious thought.

I don't doubt that the drink played some part in his weakness. In more ways than one. The group did drink a lot. The teacher always said that when a person is drunk whatever is in their heart will come out. If deep down inside they are sad or depressed the root of that depression will manifest outwardly. When someone is happy they will laugh and be merry. Others harbour anger and frustration. These are the dangerous traits. He spoke in almost therapeutic terms. Fatherly perhaps. Like karate was the means by which troubled individuals could come to terms with their inner demons. And it is. The teacher only taught a small group of students because he felt a sensei should have an understanding of their lives, what troubled them, where they've been and where they're heading.

He also spoke a lot about being drunk in another way too. Drunk on life. Drunk on karate. He would sometimes describe himself as 'The Drunkard' and I understand what he meant. When you read old texts on martial arts the writers often sound drunk. Their words poetic, vague and mysterious, hinting of double meanings, emotions and feelings. Describing the intangible with the tangible. Most of the time he really was drunk on karate.

When the three of us left the train we entered a park not far from the station. It was quieter away from the street vendors and bustle of the city; more tranquil. There was a gravel path with dim glowing lights and a gentle waterfall near a landscaped rock-wall.

"When you punch it's important to sink, hit, push and pull. All at once." We'd paused by the waterfall and my escorts had taken to coaching me in the way of punching peculiar to their style. It registered obviously but I wasn't sure of things now.

Why were they telling me this? Why had they so quickly opted to leave the bar with me? I did feel that after tonights episode it was likely I'd experience some kind of reprisal. Did they perhaps think it was going to happen sooner rather than later? I didn't doubt them. In a way I felt they were trying to do what they could to give me the best chance of coming through it.

Then one of them added worriedly. "But you mustn't say who told you. It's a secret technique!"

Actually it wasn't. It turns out that in Okinawa this is how punches are taught in a number of dojos but if you never leave the nest and look outside your own school you'd never know.

We passed a small picnic bench beneath a stylish thatched roof. A tramp was sleeping there. We left the park.

As we headed back to our dojo I wondered why this group was so closed. What made them feel that what they had was so different, so superior to anything else? And what made the members speak about their teacher like he was their father? It all felt a little stifling.

The Cult Information Centre publishes the following list of five characteristics of a cult. They are:

1. *Uses psychological coercion to recruit, indoctrinate and retain members.*
2. *Forms an elitist totalitarian society.*
3. *Its founder is self-appointed, dogmatic, messianic and charismatic.*
4. *Believes 'the end justifies the means' in order to solicit funds.*
5. *Its wealth does not benefit its members or society.*

The types of psychological techniques used by cults to recruit members include:

'*inviting the candidate to a special event or series of classes. Assign members to 'attend' to the new recruit. Place the individual in a panicky, disorientated state. Manufacture an emotional crisis and/or isolate the individual from family and friends whilst depriving them of sleep, keeping them constantly fatigued and causing them to become dependent upon the group, thus more easily persuaded.*'

Had I stumbled into a cult? At times members did appear brainwashed. At no point since getting off the plane had I heard anything not related to karate, martial arts, fighting or their 'teacher'. They spoke of nothing else. I hadn't really slept at all. I didn't even know how many days had passed since we'd arrived.

This was a 'special event', the teacher had been building it up in the months before we left England, "A once in a lifetime opportunity." He'd even said 'that' to me earlier that day, not long after rousing me and using me in that humiliating demonstration. I felt isolated. I had been since I first met them. For three months before coming to Japan I'd been allowed to train alongside them but not once was I instructed in any technique of theirs. It was odd. I'd just be told to train 'my style' next to them. They hadn't taught me a thing except for when a member made a mistake and I mentally noted the correction or scolding he was given. "Join us." Were two words I would hear more times than almost anything else. It was clear I couldn't begin to learn their style until I let go of my former training and 'Joined them'.

Yet despite the harshness of my time with them I liked the teacher. When I thought about it it was only ever him saying "join us". Given the choice I don't think The Group wanted me to join at all. Their hostility towards me always took place out of sight.

I found their techniques fascinating, their fighting ability was no nonsense and direct. In a notebook after the first time I met the teacher I wrote 'He doesn't look like a fighter but I don't know of anyone who could beat him.' I concluded with 'very charismatic'.

But the darkness was there too. The whole set up had a negative vibe running through it. He was welcoming and yet at the same time he wasn't. Acceptance was conditional.

If "Join us" was the mantra I heard most then "Kill or be killed" was the next. The 'Way of the warrior'. 'The warrior spirit'. After the incident in the bar the others staggered in late throughout the early hours. This time I felt the intensity of danger growing as they whispered and murmured in the dark.

A murderous intent was dominating my thoughts. I'd made a plan and had already prepared everything for its execution. Beneath the covers I laid fully dressed and waited.

There were several plans. For more than an hour I had thought through what was needed to blow the house sky high. Japanese homes are like tinder boxes. If a rubber hose was snagged from behind the cooker it would slowly fill the kitchen with gas. For a trigger, a match-head wedged against its lighter-strip concealed in the doorframe could set the whole thing off when someone walked in for breakfast.

But this was no good. I had no ill thoughts of any kind to my host. This was his family home and by all accounts he had been very welcoming to me. Even offering me a chance to stay longer. So for the next hour I reasoned that by 4am everyone would be back and sleeping heavy. I could stealthily pick my way to the sword-set hanging on the wall and stalk from futon to futon tracing the razor edge of the *wakizashi* across their throats as they slept in their beds.

I felt sick in the stomach. These weren't normal, rational thoughts. They felt alien and influenced by something dark and insidious. Perhaps that same oppressive vibe that seemed to resonate from this very house. Or maybe the source was The Grandmaster? 'Kill or be killed' is an old and primal meme for sure.

Nonetheless I waited until four in the morning. Then, quietly, silently, I slipped back the covers rolled away my futon and stealthily made my way to the door where my backpack was hidden beneath a rag.

The closest member to the exit, the one who'd said about the teacher 'becoming his father' stirred. He'd been watching me since I first moved and looked at me now with sympathetic eyes. He shook his head 'no' and whispered . "Don't do it. It's always hardest in the beginning."

Kill or be killed?
I say 'Live and let live.'
I left.

✷ ✷ ✷

Were they a cult? Despite scoring four out of five on the CIC criteria I'm going to say no. I am aware that members of the dojo have in the past raised money for charitable causes and maybe that is enough to exclude them from qualifying. But they were a clique and I've recounted my time with The Group for two reasons.

Firstly because this type of fanatical behaviour is not unheard of in the martial arts and people should be aware of such groups and choose to engage them with open eyes. Young men in their twenties and thirties often sense an internal divide that causes them to question their place in the world and the purpose of their existence. If the message of a charismatic individual or piece of scripture appeals to their worldview then it is natural that they will be drawn strongly into its influence. Many people sense an internal emptiness that they believe can only be filled by an external source. It can't.

Secondly, I've recounted these experiences because they are mine to do so and because the short time I spent in their company affected the future direction of my karate for years to come. I harbour no ill thoughts. Nowadays I give thanks for the experience of meeting them.

4
Furosha
'Down and out in Japan'

The moment I left that dojo a great wave of relief washed over me. I paused. Took a deep breath. Exhaled and let go.

Outside, in the early hours, Tokyo seemed relaxed. Dawn was breaking. I wandered through the streets and passed a little playground where a guy was working out. Pull-ups and stretches mainly. At this time of day the only places really open were 7-Elevens or a Japanese equivalent called Lawsons.

A road sweeper crept past. It would be about ten years before futuristic sweepers like these cleaned London streets. I walked back to the park with the waterfall from the night before.

The image of the tramp sleeping on the bench had stuck in my mind. It was a bench and picnic table with a thatched roof for shelter. He was gone now and so I sat there considering my options. Golden Week was to last another three or four days and in that time the dojo I wanted to train at would be closed so I needed to find ways to occupy my time, and my money was going to be tight. I'd lost a lot with the group and in order to make what I had left last I decided to make that bench my temporary home.

There was a loose plan in mind. Once my dojo was open I'd spend the day training there and spread the word that I was looking for somewhere to stay and see what options opened up. Back in England it would work that way. If a stranger came into the dojo who had been training in another country there would certainly be people interested in helping out. People with common interest will often help each other. If I used the park as a base and waited until Golden Week was finished I'd have just enough for food and travel.

But I felt exhausted. As I sat upon the bench a hundred 'what ifs' and doubts started to creep into my mind. The realisation that I was eighteen, alone and in a foreign land with no one to call on suddenly hit me. Maybe I should just cut my losses, go to the airport and use my open ticket to come home? I cursed and smeared away a few tears on my sleeve.

In the end it was my anger and frustration at the group that motivated me to stay. A final stand so to speak, to prove I was not wasting my time or naively following a weak 'Way'.

I walked to a nearby Lawson and bought some sweetbread and juice. Even at this early hour all the staff paused from their jobs, glanced up and greeted me the way they do in Japanese shops. Back in the park I ate my breakfast and rationally thought about what I should do. I decided I would stay. I'd relax for the rest of this week, I needed the rest. The following Monday I'd go to the *honbu*, headquarter dojo, and everything would start to fall into place.

As the machine that is Tokyo woke up the world around me came to life. On the streets the traffic increased. In the park, wardens started their rounds, and men and women in suits and skirts made their way to work.

I reasoned that my best option would be to spend the day travelling around Tokyo getting a feel for things. If I were to really make a go of it I would need to understand the city I was in and be able to at least converse with people on a basic level. Manners can carry you a long way. So before buying a travel ticket I let rush-hour pass and practiced asking basic questions to unsuspecting passersby using the little Japanese I'd learnt from tapes. It was important to get the pronunciation right with native speakers but most rushed on and seemed un-nerved at the strangeness of it all.

"Excuse me! What time is it please?" - "Where is the train station?" - "Thank you VERY much." That sort of thing.

Armed with a city map from a tourist stall and my kitbag slung over my shoulder I set out to explore the Eastern Capital; Tokyo.

In 1600 Japan witnessed one of its bloodiest and most decisive battles. Sekigahara. The result was a new military de-facto a 'Shogun' named Tokugawa Ieysasu. Although the Emperor was still recognised as the spiritual head of Japan it was the Tokugawa's who would run the show for the next 265 years.

Ieysasu established his power-base in a new capital along the eastern coast. He called it Edo, closed the country to foreign trade and within this secluded isolation the urbane 'Floating World' culture of Japan was born. The arts flourished and the city grew.

Edo was renamed Tokyo in 1868 when Imperial Forces succeeded in entering the city and exiled the remaining members of the Tokugawa family in a shift of power known as the Meiji Restoration.

In 1923 a huge earthquake occurred about fifty miles south of Tokyo causing a twelve meter high tidal wave to strike the shore. Much of Japan is mountainous and so the majority of people live in dense, crowded cities close to the coasts where the plains open up. Over 130,000 people perished, two million were made homeless and three-quarters of buildings were damaged or destroyed. Yet despite this massive destruction the 1923 earthquake enabled Tokyo to be rebuilt as a modern city. Tight winding roads were replaced with motorways and traditional one and two-storey homes replaced with concrete apartment blocks. Waste disposal and mains utilities were overhauled, hygiene improved, a new airport was built and the first underground network opened four years later.

During the mid 1990s Tokyo's population exceeded ten million. Yet despite its sheer volume of people it ran relatively smoothly. On the surface everything is clean, except the air, and all service staff, taxi drivers, train drivers, station masters and school students wear immaculate uniforms. Generally people go about their day to day lives with a sense of propriety, social belonging and without confrontation.

One of the first places I visited that day was the Budokan. Built in 1964 the Budokan, literally Hall of Martial Ways, is a huge octagonal concrete arena originally built for the judo competition of the Summer Olympics hosted that year by Japan. Its use remains predominantly for prestigious martial art events but also serves as a venue for live music concerts attracting big names under the banner 'Live at the Budokan'.

When Gichin Funakoshi first demonstrated karate on the mainland in 1922 he was invited to Tokyo by the founder of judo, Kano Jigoro who then sponsored him to teach karate at another martial art building called the Kodokan.

Funakoshi remained in Japan and instructed a number of private groups in the then little known Okinawan art of karate.

One such group included members of the Shō family which were once the former monarchy of Okinawa when the island was still the seat of power to a semi-independent 'Kingdom of the Ryukyus'. But during the Meiji Restoration the Ryukyu Kingdom found itself annexed fully into the Japanese Empire and the remaining members of the Shō family were exiled to Tokyo where they entered the peerage system of modern government.

Funakoshi's primary mentor and martial arts teacher was a man named Asato. He served as Minister of State to the last Ryukyuan king, Shō Tai, and when the family moved to Tokyo he went with them.

Asato was a master of the Okinawan martial art known as Te, a former military art once taught exclusively within the warrior clans which predated karate by over a thousand years. If Okinawa is the birthplace of karate then Te is undoubtedly its mother. Almost every book discussing the history of karate makes mention of Te in some form yet curiously it is widely believed that the art no longer exists. Some proposed that aspects of it were bizarrely preserved in the most advanced kata of karate but no one knew for sure and it seemed no one knew of any dojos or teachers teaching Te either. By all accounts it had become a 'lost art'.

Asato knew Te. In addition to its empty-hand skills he was also an expert with the sword, spear, bow and horsemanship. Oral tradition tells how he once single-handedly defeated a famous swordsman on Okinawa who had challenged him to a duel. Asato was unarmed, sitting in a garden when the challenge was proposed and rather than arrange an appropriate 'time and place' he broke from protocol, calmly stood up, and invited his challenger to attack there and then. His fame was unrivalled.

It's probable that Asato also held a position similar to that of 'Head of Intelligence' because it's said he kept detailed information on all martial art experts living in the capital at the time, recording such particulars as where they lived, what style they practised, their favourite techniques, teachers and vices. 'Know yourself and know your enemy, in one hundred battles you will not know defeat' is a titbit of Military Classics wisdom he impressed repeatedly upon the young Funakoshi.

But all that was over a hundred years ago. The world was different now. Japan was different too. On the whole, being in Tokyo in 1994 was like being in a city of the future. As a child growing up in the late seventies and eighties I imagined a future where people had pocket computers, wrist-watches that did more than just tell the time and robots that spoke to you. Tokyo was pretty much there. Yet despite the prevalence of its technological advancement something of the old world lived on too. City parks were huge and ancient, they boasted magnificent landscaped features and centuries old trees. In the Imperial Palace, which was once Tokugawa's castle, the ramparts and masonry were awe-inspiring. They echoed with the memories of a distant era and brought to life all the glory of a time when men carved their own destinies with a sword in hand.

Another train ride away I visited Kamakura. Surrounded by hills on three sides, and the waters of Sagami Bay to the south, it's easy to see why Kamakura was considered a natural fortress. During the twelfth century it served as the seat of power to the Kamakura Shogunate.

Established by the Minamoto Clan, the Kamakura Period was the blossoming flower that followed nearly 750 years of rivalry between two great families, the Minamoto and the Taira. Eventually the Minamoto succeeded in annihilating the Taira clan in a decisive sea battle, 'Dan-no-Ura'. The conflicts of the Minamoto and Taira are the subject of countless, books, comics, theatre plays, TV shows and movies in Japan. Their exploits even reach far to the south to the Ryukyu Islands and Okinawa where karate first developed.

Coming out of the station at Kamakura was like stepping back into a pocket of time. Perfectly preserved twelfth century wooden buildings had escaped both natural catastrophes and the fire bombings of WWII. People here even wore traditional clothes, kimonos and *hakama*; the split trousers worn by samurai and in contrast to the bustle of the capital, Kamakura was green and lush with nature.

Not far from the station a famous temple, the Engaku-ji, sits upon a forested hill. This is the place where Gichin Funakoshi came to study Zen Buddhism and when he died in 1957 his remains were interred here. His memorial continues to be cared for today by resident nuns in a small garden tucked away from the main flow of tourists.

By the end of the day I was shattered. And yet at the same time I felt invigorated. On the way back to my favourite park bench I accidentally got off the train one station too soon but decided to walk the short distance. It turned out it wasn't a mistake, just one of those signs from fate. Along the walk to the park I discovered an impressive modern building called the Tokyo Ayase Budokan, a full-time centre for traditional martial arts.

The reception was inviting and outside it had started to rain so I went in, removed my shoes and looked around. There were seats in the reception with videos of martial arts playing on large TV screens and corridors leading to several grand training halls.

In one such hall I saw a class of children learning judo. I'd learnt the fundamentals of judo from my father who once ran a small club in my birth-town of Bridport along the Dorset coast. By the time I was ten I wanted something with punches and kicks. Karate was a natural choice. But here in this state of the art centre the judo teacher instructed the kids how to use their 'entry grabs' as short range strikes, hooks, upper-cuts and jabs. For the first time I saw the benefit of judo, which is considered a throwing art, as an effective form of self-defence.

In another hall twice as many children were donned in full armour and screamed furious battle cries whilst charging up and down the dojo hitting each other with bamboo swords. This was *kendo*, Japanese fencing.

Upstairs, in another part of the complex, a viewing gallery overlooked a long outdoor archery range. An arrow whistled through the air and struck a straw target housed within a little wooden structure. This was *kyudo*. Way of the Bow.

Before the sword it was the bow that reigned supreme in Japanese warfare. Archery was a noble pursuit for the sons of prestigious warrior clans and on the battlefields of old two great armies would face each other while hero warriors would ride out into the open ground and issue personal challenges to heroes on the opposing side. They were lengthy affairs by anyone's standards. The challenger would first introduce himself and recount his noble pedigree and the tales of famous ancestors who had won glory in battle. If a ranked warrior on the opposing side felt so inclined then he would ride forth before the lines of foot soldiers and declare his own pedigree. These family histories could reach back hundreds of years.

Eventually they'd shoot arrows at one another. Sometimes at the defeat of one hero the losing side would withdraw from the field completely. At other times it no doubt made interesting viewing for the thousands of regular spearmen and infantrymen who'd then have to rush into a bloody melee and settle things the conventional way. Nowadays the sons of warmongers are usually closeted far away from any front-lines.

When the Mongols attempted to invade Japan in the thirteenth century the hero samurai rode out into the surf screaming their ancestral deeds at the looming fleets.

Unfortunately the Mongols didn't follow the same protocol and the lone samurai would find themselves in a rain of dark arrows.

Today, *kyudo* is not so much about 'hitting' targets as it is about unifying the mind, body and spirit; becoming one with universe. Zen. Through meditative, ritualised warfare the archer and the target transcend the confines of duality and become one. The arrow pierces the soul.

Before the bow the spear was the weapon of heroes. The kanji used to write *Bu*, meaning 'martial arts', is a depiction of two crossed spears combined with the symbol to 'cease' or 'stop'. Therefore the true meaning of the martial arts is not so much the destruction of human life but the preservation of peace.

Japan's creation myth tells the tale of a divine spear wielded by the gods. When it was dipped into the primordial oceans and lifted from the water the drops that fell from its blade formed the islands of Japan. The spear, perhaps the first refined weapon crafted by man, carried a certain prestige and with it early warrior kings wielded great power. The spear has played a crucial role in the creation of most civilisations throughout the world and here at the Ayase Budokan witnessing all of these arts gave me an insight into the spirit that is at the heart of Japan. It is an old and majestic spirit carried upon an empowering and transformative wisdom.

I left the centre deep in thought and returned to the park. It was dark now and a cool evening breeze wafted the mouthwatering scents from a local street vendor. But I was on a budget so I settled for a pre-packed teriyaki roll from Lawsons.

It might seem foolish that I took to sleeping rough in a park that week. The truth is I felt safer there than I did with my old travelling companions and I had the best nights sleep since I'd arrived in Japan. There was no fear of being assaulted, Japan has one of the lowest violent crime rates in the world. I wonder how much of that is down to the prevalence of disciplines like judo, *kendo* and *naginata* being taught in schools?

No, there was no fear of attack or even theft. The biggest concern I had was being picked up by the police for vagrancy. But in reality Japan's homeless problem, which is a big one, is conveniently ignored by the authorities. When the Japanese homeless get drunk they are more prone to laughing or sinking into depression than they are to violence. Practically every park has well maintained and regularly cleaned toilet facilities. They even have electric shaving points. Japan's *furosha*, tramps, must be amongst the cleanest in the world. I reasoned that providing I wasn't sleeping during daylight hours or making a nuisance I would remain relatively un-noticed.

5
Lost and Found
"We are all Bugeisha"

As suspected the park proved to be a good base from which to ride out the remainder of Golden Week which, as it turned out, was not one public holiday but several grouped together.

During the days I'd taken to stowing my bag out of sight behind some bushes. In the mornings, before anyone was around, I'd train in kata, stretch out and have some breakfast, read a book or write some thoughts. There were other parks around but I liked this one best. In the evenings I'd return to the Budokan in Ayase which was about a twenty minutes walk away. I had two reasons for this. First it enabled me to lose a few hours so that I wouldn't be seen loitering in the park as night crept in. Secondly I'd found a new game to play. Spot the *gaijin*.

My reasoning was that if I could meet another foreigner studying martial arts out here then it could significantly improve my situation. At the least it would give me someone to talk to. Providing that is they didn't speak Spanish or German.

On the first night there were no *gaijin* and the second night was much the same. But the third proved more fruitful. At the

back of one of the large training halls stood a tall foreign student in a black *dogi*. It looked like a style of *ju-jutsu*, literally 'soft skill/method', and sometimes the trainees attacked each other with sticks and wooden swords. After the session we chatted in the reception. His name was Craig and my luck was in. He wasn't German or Spanish, but French Canadian. I told him about my arrival with the group, sleeping in the park and the fact my dojo was closed for the week. He nodded knowingly
"It's Golden Week. Most places close down for a break."
Craig agreed I'd had quite an adventure already and wrote something down on a scrap of paper.
"Meet me at this station Saturday morning, it's out of the city so you need to look it up. There is a *taikai*, seminar, going on and there'll be other guys who've come to Japan to study martial arts. Someone will know what you should do; we are all *bugeisha*." He placed the note in my hand. It read:

'*Nodashi station. Saturday. 11am.*'

As Craig went to leave he checked his watch and shared a valuable piece of wisdom that all self-respecting *bugeisha* martial-artists doing Japan on the cheap should know. "If you go to Lawsons after 10:30pm they discount the food."

With spirits high I headed back to the park. It was still raining so I made sure I remembered the details of the note incase everything got wet. I lost my bench that night to the same tramp who first gave me the idea of sleeping rough. It didn't matter. My luck was changing. I had two teriyaki rolls for the price of one and settled on another bench nearby. It didn't have a thatched roof but it was off the ground.

By all accounts Friday was an easy day. After my morning training session I went for a walk and treated myself to breakfast somewhere else for a change. 7-Eleven. I discovered a new park with a stream flowing through it and quaint wooden bridges. Wandering about the landscaped grounds I sat and watched koi for a while before returning to the park that had been my home for the past few days. I re-packed my bag and made my way to the station one last time. Whatever happened today I would not come back here. Perhaps I was feeling a little paranoid that I'd pushed my luck with the police too far. I'm sure people were noticing me, I don't know how many other *gaijin* rough it in Japan but I imagine the number is low. Whatever would happen I'd find somewhere else to sleep tonight.

Before now I'd only travelled into the heart of Tokyo but Noda lay in the opposite direction. In some childlike way I had come to feel Japan ceased to exist beyond the metro lines I'd already familiarised myself with. Now I would have to go further out. I'd have that feeling you get when you walk somewhere new for the first time. Excited anxiety.

It took about an hour and a half on the train. When I arrived it was half ten and it looked like it was going to be a warm , sunny day. It was a little quieter out here in Noda, not as manic as other parts of Tokyo. Not quite countryside but close enough.

I waited around but there was no sign of Craig. It didn't matter. A fair few *bugeisha* were arriving and some undeniably had *rokushaku-bo*, the six foot long quarter-staffs of martial arts, as well as other types of weapons slung over their shoulders in long holdalls. To an untrained eye they might look like they were going fishing but martial artists have an eye for their own.

By quarter-past eleven the congregation slowly started to head off down the street and as Craig hadn't shown I followed at a distance. I wasn't sure where we were going. I kind of expected to arrive at another big martial arts centre like the one in Ayase, but it was better than that. A small private dojo set back a little from the road. A real dojo. I felt conspicuous. Without Craig around I had no real reason to be here, I wasn't even sure what style they learnt or whether 'outsiders' were welcome. But then, like he said, 'we are all *bugeisha*'.

The class had already started when I arrived. Students were throwing punches and taking each other down with joint locks, strikes and throws. Some rolled back to their feet and attacked again. Victors became victims and victims victors. In the open doorway, amidst everyone's shoes and kit bags, knelt a guy with his arm in a bandage. I set my own bag down outside, bowed and knelt beside him.

The first half of the session lasted over an hour. We sat in silence and watched as the sensei demonstrated strange techniques of a kind I'd never seen before. He moved with a certain fluidity. His content was serious but often he would smile warmly or cause the group to laugh with him. At times several students would attack and each time he would have them tied up in painful joint locks or walking in on the blade of their companion's weapon. Sometimes the attacks looked a little too weak to be realistic but the takedowns and throws were impressive and real enough. And, to be fair, no-one was getting smacked in the face or having bones broken whilst training.

It seemed to me that the whole fighting style had lots of deception in it. Someone would grab the sensei or throw a punch and the first thing you noticed was that he made a movement that looked as though he'd mistimed his response. Like he was 'about' to do something but, like a tottering old man it was too late. In fact, he'd already done it. No block then counter, just avoid and enter. Their power came from such seemingly odd body movements that worked to unbalance the attacker almost as soon as the attack had begun.

The dojo was also how I imagined dojo's in Japan would look. To a martial artist visiting for the first time you'd be forgiven for thinking there are dojo's on every street corner. In reality they are hard to find, often tucked away and off the beaten track. At least the ones worth finding are. On the far wall of the dojo were racks of training weapons, swords of all sizes, spears, glaives, batons and sickles on chain. There were sticks, daggers, wooden guns and more. In one corner rested a full suit of samurai armour complete with an impressive helmet, shin guards and gloves. None of this was ornamental or for show. They were all battered and well used.

During the break I spoke with my fellow spectator. His name was Sasha and he was meant to be training but had injured his wrist the day before and needed to rest it. Sasha came from Croatia and was living out here learning the martial art. The style was called Bujinkan Taijutsu and the sensei's name was Dr Masaaki Hatsumi.

Hatsumi holds the rank of *Soke* and claims to be the 34th Grandmaster of the Togakure school. As I understand it Taijustu is just one of nine branches or 'specialisations' taught within the Bujinkan syllabus. However unlike other martial arts the style teaches a very diverse range of subjects because in addition to empty hand and weaponry trainees can also learn geography, meteorology, fighting whilst swimming, herbalism, fieldcraft, psychology, disguise, weapon concealment, impersonation and other skills well suited to espionage.

The Bujinkan have spies. Or rather, they are spies. As well as assassins, smugglers, infiltrators and saboteurs. This is because Togakure ryu is a school of *ninjitsu* that claims its origins reach back to the time of the Minamoto and Taira conflicts of the twelfth century.

The founder, Daisuke Nishina, was a member of the Minamoto clan and after a big rebellion he retreated to the forested hills of the Kii peninsular to save his family. There, the story goes, he met a Chinese monk living in political exile who taught him a subtle martial art which became the root of *ninjitsu*, the art of 'stealing in'.

Historically, *ninjas* and *shinobi's* would be employed by samurai armies to infiltrate and create spy networks, gather intelligence on castle structures, report on troop numbers and sabotage plans. As well as assassinate rival generals, broker deals or conduct guerrilla warfare. When Tokugawa Iyesasu set his capital at Edo in the seventeenth century he drew upon *ninja's* to create his secret police.

Today Hatsumi sensei teaches people from all over the world and has been contracted to train agents from several Intelligence and Special Forces. The Bujinkan banner swells with members but to me its internal structure always seemed a little loose compared with other schools, so who can tell what will happen to the quality of its techniques in the future.

During the break I told Sasha about my situation and how I'd come to be there that morning. He contemplated for a while and we watched the second half of the session. Afterwards he turned to me and said "I live close-by. If you're interested I have a spare room you could rent." This sounded like something worth considering so after the *taikai* we walked to the apartment, which really wasn't very far away, and it was big by Japanese standards.

The front door opened into a large kitchen area with a raised floor and a small bathroom on the opposite side. Then there were two rooms floored with traditional *tatami* straw mats. Tatami are about three-feet by six and a standard measurement in Japanese buildings. It was perfect and at once felt like something was really coming together, something more akin to how I imagined my Japanese adventure would be. "Look, if you like you could stay tonight and decide in the morning. It seems crazy to go and sleep in a park."

And that's how I came to set some roots down and concentrate on my training in Japan. And such is the hospitality of genuine martial artists, or *bugeisha*. Yes combat-efficiency needs to be there, perhaps even the notion of 'kill or be killed' on some level, but what really matters is the ability to get along with others. To share and grow. Mutual respect for others built on an understanding of differences while at the same time recognising the things that make us the same. No 'one' martial art style is better than another it's different strokes for different folks. They can all have value providing they are taught in a positive and creative way.

In the apartment I had the smaller of the two rooms. It was only four and a half *tatami* but it was home. In a cupboard I found a bundle of bedding including a futon mattress and large, almost antique, *dotera*, a sort of patchwork quilted winter kimono that was so big I could sleep in it.

Sasha became my mentor for all things to do with living in Japan. He taught me to shop on certain days when the supermarkets slashed their prices, how to use the international phone-booths and how to use ninja psychology to cut in line when Iranian businessmen were hogging the public phones to do their business; whatever 'that' was.

Once a week we would hire videos from a local store and we played them on a machine that we pulled from the bins. Most appliances in the house came from local bins. In Japan during the mid-nineties you could pretty much find any gadget you wanted from other people's rubbish. We had a TV, radio, cd-player and rice-cooker all collected from refuse not because they were broken but because newer models had come on the market and the Japanese are superstitious of second-hand goods.

Noda is an industrialised area that once served as a way-station for trade entering Edo along the Edogawa river. Not many have heard of the town but most people have heard of Kikoman Soy Sauce. If you buy a bottle of soy-sauce that is shaped with a bell-bottom and capped with a red top then chances are it is produced by Kikoman and it might have been brewed in Noda. The whole town smelt of soy-sauce due to the fact of several large refinery plants there. Noda is also famous for its rice-crackers which make acceptable boxed gifts to give to Japanese friends when you visit them.

As our friendship grew we would often eat our dinner together and talk about martial arts and future plans late into the night. My arrival in Japan had seemed like a violent Typhoon but now it seemed the storm was clearing and things were settling down.

6
Knock Knock
"I've come to learn karate."

At last Golden Week drew to an end and so the next day I phoned the *honbu* dojo of Kanazawa sensei's 'SHOTOKAN INTERNATIONAL KARATE FEDERATION' and wrote down the times I could train. The problem was that the dojo was now a two hour train ride away from where I was staying. Also, I knew that that Kanazawa sensei was teaching abroad at the time so I figured that in addition to training at the *honbu* I could try to find some other Shotokan dojo's that were closer to home.

In the back of an instructional book written by Kanazawa there is a list of addresses in Japanese. I assumed they were dojo's and so asked the checkout-girl in the local supermarket if she could translate the 'closest' one to Noda. It was an hour away. That afternoon I rode down to the station caught a train back towards Tokyo and set out to find it.

There is a rumour that street addresses in Japan are not numbered in sequential order but more closely to the order in which a house was built. I don't know if that is true or not but it seemed plausible because I must have spent two hours wandering up and down streets looking for that address. I'd stop to ask directions but ultimately ended up going in circles. Nothing resembled anything like a dojo whether it be commercial or private. Reluctantly I returned home.

The next afternoon I tried again. One house in particular kept drawing me back. It was set away from a gated stone wall with an intercom buzzer but it didn't match the image of a dojo in my mind so I kept on walking. After a while I stopped in the garden of a nearby shrine and practiced a kata. A 'temple kata'. *Jion*.

At that time in my training I enjoyed the practice of kata immensely, I found it deeply rewarding on a personal level and a good workout too. In kata you train alone but teachers would often labour the importance of 'imagining' your opponent as you performed each technique in sequence. This helps to bring the sequence to life and perhaps is one of the things that makes karate different to dance.

Yet despite the constant reminder teachers gave to 'imagine your opponent' instruction in what each technique was actually doing was often ignored. In Shotokan there were no 'official' *bunkai* - you made it up in your head. Most of the time you kept it there. In the regimented dojo students didn't ask questions, they just did what their sensei told them to do.

Nowadays a lot of Shotokan trainees try to find *bunkai*, fighting applications, in the movements of their kata, but before the nineties they didn't really exist. Funakoshi never taught any and Itosu, the teacher that taught him kata, never taught any either. The whole time I was in Japan the subject never came up in the dojo.

Sometimes, like on a seminar, a senior Japanese instructor might suggest what a particular movement in a kata was meant to be doing. Most of the time they required far too many variables to be 'just right' to be considered realistic. For example the aggressor 'had' to attack with a right-handed corkscrew punch and lead with his right foot forward for the predetermined defence to work. Usually he would have to leave the punch out so that the attack could be fantastically defeated with a dynamic, and usually, 'over the top' response.

In reality, as a defender, you simply couldn't guarantee that kind of conformity from an attacker hell bent on causing you harm. The exercise was always a little pointless.

There in the quiet grounds of the shrine I'd taken to rehearsing kata in sets of three. One repetition at medium pace, then one fast and the last very slow. I would try to make the slow version last more than a few minutes. It helped to clear the mind.

When I finished, I rested on a small bench and contemplated the movements of *Jion*. I also wondered why I couldn't find the dojo. A black cat laced through my legs and purred.

Jion is the last of the original kata that Funakoshi introduced into his karate style. Today Shotokan has twenty six kata but originally Funakoshi only brought fifteen from Okinawa. These were the five *Heian* kata's, three *Tekki* forms, *Bassai*, *Kwanku*, *Empi*, *Gankaku*, *Jutte*, *Hangetsu* and *Jion*.

Each one teaches a different range of techniques and attitudes and Funakoshi's original intention was that students would be 'prescribed' the kata's best suited to their physique and current understanding of karate. Not everyone would have learnt all fifteen kata.

Of course once the style became hugely popular this individualised approach to teaching was no longer feasible. It needed to be standardised. Over the years the movements of the forms were simplified, extended and altered into their current style. Part of the reason this occurred is because of the distinct absence of *bunkai*. Had Funakoshi taught the combative applications of the kata then it's less likely the movements would have been altered much at all.

He didn't teach them because of the large number of students now learning karate and his fear that the art might find destructive expression in a pointless street brawl. In his eyes the karate he was teaching, just as his teacher Itosu had introduced years earlier on Okinawa, was for the development of health and character. Not for fighting. The true student of the art would unlock the real meanings of the kata through diligent self-practice and introspection. But they would not learn them in a class although their meanings were passed down orally.

Perhaps Funaksohi never envisioned the radical changes that were to follow in his absence. Then again. Perhaps he did. In the opening pages of his book Karate-Dō Kyohan a poem, brushed by the author, reads:

'To search for the old is to understand the new.
The old, the new
This is a matter of time.
In all things man must have a clear mind.
The Way:
Who will pass it on straight and true?'

The cat sauntered off into the peaceful grounds of the shrine.

A person raised in Europe or America might superstitiously believe that when a black cat crosses their path it is an ominous sign of ill fortune. In England, as in Japan, people say the opposite is true. It's all about perception. What seems like one thing to one person can seem like something else to another. In all things it is best to keep an open mind.

Karate's literal translation is 'empty hand'. In the English language this has crudely come to mean 'unarmed combat' but the kanji for '*kara*', empty, carries a certain zen-like notion. 'Empty' is the mind of the one who studies the way of the 'hand'. An empty mind is one not clouded by pre-conceived images or judgements. In karate we liken it to the surface of a polished mirror - so clean that it only reflects what is before it and nothing of itself.

These past two days I had assumed I was looking for a dojo, a hall or training centre of some sort, but perhaps the dojo was at someone's home? I smiled, shook my head at my thoughtlessness and headed back to the gate in the wall.

"I've come to learn karate." I announced to the lady's voice that answered the intercom. "Karate student".

"Ah! Hai!" came her response. After a while I heard her footsteps approaching and the slide of the bolt as she opened the gate. A little surprised at my arrival she bowed and beckoned me in to the garden. I couldn't see a hall or gymnasium but the garden and the house were in a traditional style. The house itself was the biggest on the street and constructed in timber with traditional craftsmanship. I wondered how old it was and what miraculous fate it had to survive all the bombings of WWII.

"Sensei is busy in a meeting. Please. Come and wait."

She led me into the main entrance of the house to a small waiting room with a wooden floor and low table. Realising at once that I had made a terrible faux pas I burned with embarrassment. Turning up to a sensei's house without an appointment was certainly not in accordance with Japanese etiquette. I couldn't be sure how this was going to play out.

Ten minutes later I heard two men saying goodbye in the hallway and the front-door close. A discussion between a man and the women began outside the room and I shrank with the awkwardness of it all. When he entered he did so with a bemused but friendly smile.

"Hello?"

I bowed and introduced myself in text book style. Announcing that I was a student of karate. That I had arrived from England and had come to learn.

He was tall by Japanese standards, with a round face and short moustache. The top of his head was bald and as he took a seat opposite he stroked his jaw in contemplation.

"Why are you here?" He asked.

"*Watashi-wa karate no gakusei desu*! - I'm a karate student!"

He looked me over and smirked with the bizarreness of it all and asked again in English.

"Yes. But 'why' are you here? How did you find me?"

Reaching into my small backpack I took out my well travelled copy of Kanazawa's book and opened it to the page of addresses with his underlined. Of course this only half answered his question because 'why' was his the only address underlined? At length I succeeded in explaining that I'd come to train at the *honbu-dojo* but was living out in Noda. He nodded and seemed to half understand.

An interview began. Sort of.
"What is your name? How old are you? Where do you live?" Mostly I could answer in Japanese. Our conversation became a mix of the two.
"You are eighteen? Where are you parents?"
"England." He frowned with confusion.
"Who are you with?"
"No one. I have come to Japan to learn karate."
"You come alone?"
"Hai!" Later I felt my age and tenacity played strongly in my favour and at length he held his hand up and nodded.
"OK. What grade are you?"
"Shodan."
"Black belt? You are black belt?" He looked at my bag
"Do you have dōgi?"
"Hai!" I opened the bag and showed him my uniform.

He smirked with an approving nod and then turned serious. "OKAY. I am Mr Sawada. Tonight you train with me. My dojo. Then tomorrow you come here. 9am. I take you to *honbu-dojo*. Understand?"
I nodded and bowed my head. Then he continued.
"After tomorrow. You no come here again. You only train *honbu*." I felt a little sorry at that but reasoned it was fair enough. I had intruded on his hospitality and figured he wasn't looking for any new students. At least tonight I could start training with others who practised the same style as I did.
About twenty minutes later we drove in his car to a small local hotel where a wooden building sat just inside the grounds. This was his dojo. A private dojo.
It was a little dusty. Large enough for classes although I doubted that many regular sessions were taking place here. It had a beautiful hardwood floor and one wall with large mirrors that could be closed off with wooden shoji screens. A few free-

weights were stacked in a corner, along with something like an antique cross-trainer from the sixties, a wooden *makiwara* and a sand-filled punch-bag which felt like it had long turned to concrete.

I changed into my gi and started limbering up waiting for the others to arrive. About ten minutes passed before the door opened again and when it did in came a Japanese student my age. He had a stocky build and a flop of dark hair that he swept back with his hand. He paused at once and looked at me as if I were from Mars. Mr Sawada spoke with him and introduced us.

"This is my student. His name is Masakazu."

We bowed hello and then Mr Sawada said. "Lets begin."

It turned out Masakazu was Mr Sawada's private student. The son of a close friend, he was studying for university. He intended to become a doctor. Mr Sawada was in his mid-forties and, in the year Masakazu and I were born, our teacher won First Place in an international karate tournament. At the time of my arrival in Japan he was a 7th dan black-belt, having trained directly under Kanazawa and was now the Chief Manager of the Japanese Karate Team.

The warm up was intense. Four sets of fifty press-ups, sit-ups, front snap kicks and reverse punches, left and right sides. All in *kihon* basic style. Then combinations of front kick, round-house, crescent, turning back kick, side-snap followed by a side thrust kick. Twenty times over, the length of the dojo back and forth.

Then the lesson began. My legs quivered with fatigue as we held front-stance and Mr Sawada broke down the fundamental attacks most suited for sparring. Front-jab, reverse punch and front snap kick. This kind of training was all about not giving up and perfecting technique. The sweat streamed down our faces. The mirrors fogged. Our faces were flushed red and we struggled to keep our breath. My punch was corkscrewing too wide, Masakazu's hips were too high.

Silently we had united through our determined spirit under Sawada's relentless *"mou-ichido!"* 'one more time!' Always 'one more time'. I would not give up. Ever. And it was clear that my training partner felt the same. We must have performed close to two-thousand punches and kicks that session. The inside of my wrists chaffed and split upon the sides of my white gi as I worked hard to prevent my elbows going wide whilst punching. The blood peppered upon the cotton and my heart felt like it was going to pound out of my chest. Then, without rest, Mr Sawada announced "*Kumite.*"

First we were drilled in the fundamental fighting postures of attack and defence before free-style "*jiyu kumite*". This was Mr Sawada's expertise and Masakazu was clearly his student.

Finally the pace started to ease down. Had someone have forewarned me I'd have doubted it was possible to train in all we had that session. And it wasn't over yet.

"Kata."

We performed a basic level kata first. *Heian Sandan.* Then the next two in the *Heian* set. Afterwards we demonstrated *Tekki-Shodan* then *Bassai Dai.*

"Do you know *Kanku Dai?*" Sawada asked.

"Yes sensei" He raised his brow and glanced to Masakazu who was now catching his breath and watching from the sideline.

"Please show. *Kanku Dai.*"

"Hai."After *Kanku Dai* I was quizzed on my knowledge of other kata.

"*Jion?*"

"Hai."

"*Hangetsu?*"

"Hai."

"*Gankaku?* You know *Gankaku?* Please show. *Gankaku.*"

Truth be told, at that time I could perform any kata from the Shotokan set. Perhaps some teachers would consider it bad form to learn kata beyond your grade level. Technically I was still only *Shodan*; first black belt. But I had been training a long time. Karate was my life. At school I was never interested in sports. Even today I don't regard karate as a sport. It's just something I do.

My sensei back in England knew the entire Shotokan syllabus like the back of his hand. He was a *sandan*, third level black-belt. He coached me in kata one at a time until I could perform the entire sequence naturally. It was the part of training I enjoyed the most. I don't recommend learning so many forms today though. For one it is not necessary. Funakoshi's original set of fifteen is more than enough. Perhaps even too many.

Another two kata's in and I was exhausted. Finally the session naturally wound down into conversation.

"What grade are you?" Sawada asked with a frown.

"*Shodan* sensei!"

"*Shodan?*" He exclaimed with confusion. He shook his head and struggled to explain his thoughts. Masakazu tried to interpret but it was too difficult. At length Mr Sawada asked in child like terms.

"You are black belt yes?" I nodded. "But what is your rank?" Again I responded "*Shodan.*" It seemed things weren't going well at all. There was much head shaking and Mr Sawada and Masakazu spoke too quickly for me to gauge what was being discussed. Now my training partner tried another approach. "How long you train karate?" I couldn't think of the Japanese word for years so I held up eight fingers. This brought approving nods and raised brows. Then Mr Sawada said. "You are *nidan!*" second black-belt. I faltered and shook my head no. In the morning I was being taken to the *honbu* and didn't want to be introduced there as anything beyond my grade level. I couldn't understand why this was becoming an issue. I tried to protest and explain once more but then he turned very serious and cut the air with his hand.

"NO! You are *nidan*! Anyone ask your grade, you say NIDAN! You tell them. Mr Sawada your teacher. You are *nidan!*" He nodded firmly and looked to Masakazu, who nodded approvingly. They both looked to me. I nodded cautiously and bowed. Did I just get graded?

"Tomorrow you come to my house. 9am. I take you to *honbu dojo*. You train there." I nodded some more. It seemed all I could really do. The soles of my feet were burning from the friction of the workout on the hardwood floor and I'm not sure what was stopping me from collapsing in a heap.

"After you train at *honbu* you come here. I teach you. Understand? In the evenings you train here."

This was more than I could have hoped for. The session was over. I felt on fire and we got changed. Mr Sawada left and Masakazu walked me back to the train station. Along the way he asked me about London and my travels. Naturally I invited him to visit one day and once we reached the station he cycled off home and I caught the train back to Noda. It was late, the stars were out and the cool air was a welcome reward after the gruelling session. When I got back Sasha wanted to hear all about my training but it would have to wait. I was shattered and had an early start. He set an alarm for me while I showered, ate some bread and fell into a deep sleep.

7
Finding Balance
"Stand bow. Not bow. BOW!"

As Spring gave way to the wet season Japan became a bloom of rich growth. Out in Noda there were plenty of green fields but the sky was often overcast. At the back of our apartment the doors opened onto a small wooden ledge and postage stamp of grass. Usually I would use a concrete fence pillar as a *makiwara*, sometimes I'd practice balancing on one leg and kicking with an umbrella in hand. Eventually the rains washed away the fallen cherry blossoms and cleared for a hot and humid summer.

Training in karate is a cleansing process. During my days in Japan I would travel to the *honbu dojo* in the Kugahara district of Tokyo. Sessions were gruelling but not destructive. Everyone was pushed to their limits but the sensei's were always aware of each students' ability and inner strengths. The core teaching staff had mostly come from the university clubs and the content of each session usually revolved around the three aspects of *kihon*, *kumite* and *kata*. Instruction was always in Japanese but there were often times when someone present could translate a specific teaching point into English if needed.

The atmosphere at Kanazawa's dojo was always friendly and throughout the classes in the day many faces would become familiar to me. The feeling was like one of an extended family. Doctors, office workers, college students, CEO's and visitors from abroad, all working in Japan, training together, united by karate.

Before travelling to Japan I'd heard horror stories that 'westerners' were singled out and targeted in the dojo's by hardline patriotic students looking to prove a point. It never happened here. Perhaps it was the horror story of a former time, during the sixties and seventies perhaps, when my teachers had come on their own pilgrimages. To me everyone at the dojo seemed genuinely interested to meet new visitors and to hear stories about their homelands and travels.

With my introduction from Mr Sawada I was afforded the opportunity to spend significant time with the instructors of the dojo Nobuaki, Tanaka, Suzuki and Ichihara. On occasion I'd travel with them to other classes around the city too. Nobuaki Kanazawa is tall, athletic and light-hearted, his technique crisp, fast and clean; as you might expect it would be being the eldest son of a world-class teacher. Nobuaki had a great sense of humour and was a pleasure to spend time with. His father, Hirokazu Kanazawa is *kancho*, he heads the whole organisation.

Born in 1931 Kanazawa trained under Masatoshi Nakayama, a driving figure in the standardisation of Shotokan, but he also had the opportunity to train with Gichin Funakoshi. The year after Funakoshi's death the Japan Karate Association broke with protocol and hosted the First All Japan Karate Championship. The move caused a rift within the karate world that ultimately led to two groups forming from Funakoshi's original students. One group, headed by Shigeru Egami, continued the masters teachings and opposed the introduction of competition. They took the name Shotokai. The other group, the JKA continued to develop the style into a modern budō that is the Shotokan style of today.

In 1957 Kanazawa entered the first All Japan Karate Championship but broke his arm in the lead up to the event.

Feeling disheartened he was about to retract his entry when his mother said to him. "In karate are you taught to only use your hands? Do you not also learn to use your legs and body too?" Indeed you do. With renewed spirit Kanazawa entered the competition and went on to win first place, literally single-handed with one arm in a sling. Today his SKIF organisation has affiliated dojos across 130 countries and he spends much of the year traveling the world teaching courses.

In the evenings I would return from the *honbu* to Mr Sawada's dojo where I'd receive another couple of hours private instruction in *kumite* before finally heading back to Noda.

Some days I'd stay close to home to train by myself or do the same at Sawada's dojo which he had given me access to. There were three 'spaces' I had for personal training. A short walk away from the apartment, along a narrow path through paddy-fields, was an old Buddhist shrine and within the grounds was a stage area beneath a tiled roof which became my 'rainy day' and 'moonlight' training space. On other days I'd jog the mile distance to the edge of the Edogawa river and train in the sun along its banks.

One day Masakazu and I cleaned the dojo from top to bottom, using rags and hot water to wipe down the walls and floor and old newspapers for the mirrors and windows. I liked to train there the most. It was a perfect space quietly tucked away from the manic bustle of Tokyo. I could go to that dojo to meditate and focus upon my personal training anytime I liked.

Training alone I'd usually focus on kata. I reasoned I was getting enough of a fitness workout from the regular classes at the *honbu* and under Mr Sawada's guidance my *kumite* was radically improving. I was leaner now. More flexible and faster. Yet all the while something inside me felt empty. Instinctively I came to feel there was something missing in my training. In Shotokan generally. I suspect others have felt this nagging feeling too. The words of Funakoshi's poem lingered in my mind *'To search for the old is to understand the new.'*

Coupled with the contradictions of his advice for trainees to 'become not hard but soft' Funakoshi's karate seemed juxtaposed to the style currently being taught in mainstream dojos, which was, by all accounts, very hard in nature. Was I now searching for the old to make sense of the new? And if so, where would I begin my search?

Funakoshi's writings suggested that everything was there in the kata. That the practice of kata itself should not simply entail the memorising of movements for movements sake, but that the meanings of the movements themselves must be understood.

'Once a form has been learnt it must be practiced repeatedly until it can be applied in an emergency, for knowledge of just the sequence of a form in karate is useless.'

My experiences in Japan had so far exposed me to a spectrum of ideas and concepts. Not just about karate but martial arts in general. I turned now to the practice of kata and delved deeply into the rabbit hole. Although my training in *kumite* was improving I knew in my heart that it as nowhere near the calibre of the group I first arrived in Japan with. Shotokan was for sport but for me karate was much more than that. Was I looking for fighting ability though, or was I seeking perfection of technique? I certainly wasn't seeking fame or trophies from competition so I decided I would concentrate on just a few kata and focus on 'seeing' the *bunkai* applications within them.

I chose forms from Funakoshi's original set of fifteen; *Kanku Dai*, *Empi* and *Gangaku*. For me these three forms represented a range of techniques suited to my natural build and fighting style. Instead of practising many kata superficially I pulled these three apart and contemplated them deeply. Funakoshi's original kata had been modified since he first introduced them from Okinawa all those years ago. At that time however I had no idea as to what movements had been changed and no access to older versions of the forms to compare them with.

I knew that he didn't practise in the low stances so widely used today. Front stance, back stance and side stance were all performed much higher. They were more natural. Therefore I started to practice in these higher stances too.

In the UK if your stance wasn't long or deep enough a sensei would likely crack down heavy on you but here, in Japan, at Kanazawa's dojo, I often saw people of different ages and abilities training in stances of varying heights. And they didn't get criticised for it. I reasoned that there are three 'frames' upon which Shotokan techniques could be performed. High, medium and low. Most training was in the medium to low category but these stances were often too stressful for some of the older practitioners to perform well. They naturally used higher stances instead and this was never looked down upon in class providing they still applied the correct body dynamics required.

During these private workouts I used the higher frame of which afforded greater manoeuvrability within the kata themselves. But only in private. Whenever I was in a class or being instructed by Mr Sawada I would return to the deeper stances they expected to see. I used their training sessions to maintain strong basic form and explored the changes I was making in my own personal training.

Of course it's naive to think that simply adopting a higher stance immediately equates to 'training the old way'. It doesn't. But it did at least provide a model upon which to make further explorations.

*

"Okay, here. Stop. Throw anchor.
Good. Stand bow.
Not bow. Bow!
Up!"

"What, up front?"
"Make block ...learn balance... balance key... if balance good, karate good. Everything good."

It was movie night at the apartment. A classic. *The Karate Kid*. Right now Mr Miyagi has taken Daniel-san fishing and is getting him to practice his techniques whilst standing on the bow of the small rowing boat. Daniel-san starts to question his teacher about karate and fighting.

"You mean there were times when you were scared to fight?"
"Always scared. Miyagi hate fighting."
"But you like karate."
"So?"
"Karate's fighting, you train to fight."
Miyagi frowns "That what you think?"
Daniel-san falters. "um... no."
"Then why train?"
"So I won't have to fight." Miyagi smiles and nods approvingly. "Miyagi have hope for you."

I smile because earlier that week I was on a train with Mr Sawada and he was teaching me about balance. We were on a trip into the city and although there were seats available he beckoned me to stand like him near the doors.
"Stand like this. Good for karate. Good for balance."

We call it *shizentai-dachi*; natural ready stance. Standing with your feet about a shoulders width apart it's the first stance you learn in the dojo. The knees should be pliable. Not rigid but not too relaxed either. Just 'ready'. The weight is centred into the *hara* and your shoulders are dropped. From this position you should be able to respond instantly to an attack. When it is practiced in the dojo the stance is quite rigid. Sometimes teachers will come and kick your legs, or punch your stomach to see if you are standing strong. But here, on the train, it was different. Mr Sawada was showing a more natural way to adopt *shizentai-dachi*. It was closer to surfing or skateboarding, you had to be relaxed so as to feel the movement of the train and keep your balance. We rode the line like this for a few stops and then got off.
"Always find ways to practice karate every day." Now he was walking up the steps of the platform using just the balls of his feet.

I was starting to see that karate was really all about balance. Not just physical balance like standing on the train or not being swept to the ground by an opponent, but mental and spiritual balance too. In order to defeat an opponent you have to break their physical balance with a kick, strike or throw but there's more. Don't we also speak of mental balance? Concentration. Sometimes we use techniques to break the opponent's concentration, to distract or confuse them with feints, and setup attacks. Then there is spiritual balance. In karate we might shatter an opponent's spiritual composure with a strong *kiai* or stern gaze. But before we can even begin to succeed over others we first need our own mental, physical and spiritual balance. In the Chinese Classics it says that in ancient times warriors first made themselves invincible. This didn't mean through reliance on external devices, like European knights attempted with armour and weaponry, but through inner strength cultivated through focussed mental composure and physical ability. In the Far East ancient warriors first made themselves strong by finding inner balance. The link between spiritual fortitude and martial arts in the Far East reaches back to ancient India.

Another time, in the company of Mr Sawada, the subject of balance came up again.

"Balance is very important."

We had just finished another intense workout. It was a muggy evening and my sweat soaked gi had been annoyingly dragging across my extremely sunburnt legs. Earlier that day I'd fallen asleep by the edge of the Edo river on the count of generally feeling exhausted as a result of the heavy training sessions. Mr Sawada looked at my lobster red legs with a knowing grin.

"You are young and karate is good for you. But also it's very hard." As I tried to pull on my jeans he continued.

"If you always train hard then karate not good for you. You will be tired. Your muscles will become stiff. You should find other ways to balance your hard training."

This was very similar to something Kanazawa had said too. Kanazawa sensei had discussed that he felt the intensity of his early training had taken a heavy toll upon his health. That is why he took up Tai Chi under Ming Shi Yang. Even his teacher, Nakayama, had studied Tai Chi and endorsed its benefits to health and vitality. Was this another facet missing from Shotokan training? Had the youthful enthusiasm of modern karate's first exponents like Kanazawa and others such as Asai, Nishiyama and Egami played a detrimental role in their later years? In their youth they were lean hardbodies with ripped muscles layered upon muscles. But as they aged all of them sought ways to soften their karate and none can honestly be said to have aged gracefully.

When the JKA directed Shotokan towards sport Shigeru Egami broke away to form the Shotokai. His karate became increasingly softer and more fluid. Almost unrecognisably so some might argue. Kanazawa had also started to introduce aspects of Tai Chi and yoga into his warmups. It was also obvious that many of the teachers I were meeting recognised a clear link between fighting arts and healing arts combined.

The karate master of the dojo I first stayed at upon arrival was a practitioner of shiatsu, a form of Japanese bodywork that applies pressure to specific points on the body to release stress and tension so as to restore natural health and vitality.

Then there was The Grandmaster. He was skilled in acupuncture, a Chinese therapy which claims to re-direct pain and harmonise the flow of intrinsic energy, '*ki*', to nurture people back to health. Even the ninjas in Noda studied herbalism. My flatmate also practiced traditional massage, bone-setting and medicine.

In a different way Shotokan was also attracting members of the medical world. Mr Sawada's work was related to modern medicine as was my training partners father. Masakazu himself was studying to become a doctor and there were other doctors in the classes at the *honbu* too.

It seemed clear that knowledge of the natural healing arts led to a greater understanding and awareness of the body. Knowledge of how to strike at anatomical weak-spots empowered smaller individuals to significantly increase their chances against larger or more numerous attackers.

One day Mr Sawada announced that he was going away for two weeks for an operation on his knee. It was a story being told to me by so many of the more matured karate-ka I'd encountered over the years that it really started to drive home the issue of destructive training. Was Shotokan really doing any of us any favours? I took the opportunity of my teacher's absence to ease down on the harsher aspects of my training and investigate ways to 'balance' my karate. I joined a local group practicing Tai Chi in a park and enrolled in the study of shiatsu therapy.

It seemed that in no time at all the Tai Chi training had a very positive effect on my karate. Within three months my lung capacity increased and I found I was able to control my breathing far more efficiently during *kumite* practice. I also wasn't getting out of breath as quickly as my opponents did. The slow moving techniques also helped to soften my muscles and my seniors berated me far less about 'dropping my shoulders'. During my personal training I applied the lessons of Tai Chi to the slow repetitions of my kata practice. I discovered that I was gaining greater awareness of every minute aspect of my techniques and when the transmission from one movement to the next seemed 'juddered' or not smooth, then I knew this was the weak-spot of that particular motion. I would then isolate those movements to practice them over and over until they felt completely natural.

Tai Chi also helped to calm the mind and increase my sensitivity. In time I gained greater awareness of the subtle 'tell tale' signs that preceded my opponent's attacks. With practice I found I was able to remain relaxed in sparring, unflustered by attempts to feint or distract so that I could directly enter at the moment an opponent changed their guard or made some careless movement. It was as though I could sense, their thoughts had changed and in 'that' precise moment could enter and succeed.

The shiatsu training was equally beneficial but in other ways. It taught me a great deal about the body and its internal functions, about how tight muscles could be released through applying the appropriate pressure to key points or '*tsubo*'. Many of these *tsubo* correlated exactly to the 'vital points' in the karate texts of old and came hand in hand with the knowledge of how to seize or strike them to cause injury. Several years later shiatsu was to become my profession and I eventually specialised in treating martial art injuries, back pain, sleeping problems and relieving the symptoms of stress related illnesses.

Of course all of this took many years of training to cultivate. In the weeks Mr Sawada was away my understanding of them was very limited but my interest definitely sparked.

Funakoshi used to say that the practice of karate was primarily for the benefit of health and that self-defence was secondary to this. I wanted my karate to be more than just a means of developing personal health and self-defence. I wanted it to provide a means for helping others do the same too. In this way I started to reason that I was seeking a karate that was complete and that in order to have it I needed to find the origins of Funakoshi's art. Ultimately I realised that sooner or later I would have to start looking outside of Shotokan, but where?

8
The Old Man in the park
"Shotokan didn't used to be like this."

Friday. Early morning at the *honbu*. A visitor from America is translating the elderly Japanese man at the front of the class for my benefit.

"Shotokan didn't used to be like this."

In order to make this session I had spent the week at a local *ryokan*, traditional inn, just ten minutes walk away from the dojo. I wanted to know what the content was like in these early classes because my usual two-hour commute from Noda meant I could never get to them in time.

The Old Man was not the scheduled teacher of the class. That was Ichihara sensei. But about ten minutes ago Ichihara finished warming us up and teaching some basics when he turned and bowed to the Old Man training next to me and asked him to demonstrate a point. The whole thing had an air of Japanese protocol to it.

He was stocky, with a rounded chest and happy face. I'm not sure of his age but perhaps he was in his late seventies. I regret I never learnt his name on the count of being swept up by the things he was saying and demonstrating. Perhaps, when I share this you'll forgive me this oversight. I remember him fondly as the 'Old Man' with an honorific tone and none of the derogatory implications of age implied in the West. He was old and wise, and a little playful too.

Before the session had started I'd seen him kicking one of the concrete pillars holding up the ceiling with his shin. Despite his age he had real power and a solid build. What struck me first about his teaching style was how 'down to earth' and informal it was compared to other teachers. He smiled and had an enjoyable presence about him, yet despite this, when the class was handed over, the younger trainees seemed a little disenchanted. I guess they preferred a hard blasting workout before heading off to university and this sensei took a different approach.

As he started to talk I became hooked.

"When he was younger he trained with Funakoshi; during the early days." The American was leaning in and quietly translating for me so as not to disrupt the class. My eyes widened.

The first thing he had us do was perform the technique *age-uke*, upper block. Fists clenched and arms bent above our heads he proceeded to lift a punchbag from its mounting and walk down the ranks of trainees using it like a mallet to test the strength of our blocks. Everyone's *age-uke* failed and the heavy end of the punchbag hit our heads.

"Funaksohi would teach like this."

Now he had the class perform *age-uke* with an open hand curling only the smallest finger tightly as if it were in a fist; the remaining fingers were held as straight as possible. Again the punchbag came round but this time no one's technique failed. The punchbag just fell upon our forearms and it was almost effortless to keep it there.

"When you close your fist, always tighten the smallest finger. Very important." He watched us perform *age-uke* until he was satisfied we understood and then demonstrated the same technique again, but this time not as a block, but a punch.

Having re-hung the punchbag he showed the full force of this strike with impressive results. His largest knuckles struck into the bag firmly and it shook to its base like a snake leaving a clean impact crater. Next he used *age-uke* to defend against an opponent's attack. Not in the usual way by sweeping their attacking arm upwards but by simply stepping in and using the technique as a punch to either the temple, jaw or throat. The shape of the strike meant it easily went around and over a persons usual defence. It was more circular and finished with a curious quiver from his waist that enabled a great amount of power to be transferred into the target.

Then front kick, *maegeri*. This too differed from the usual version taught in class. The Old Man demonstrated all techniques from what I had then taken to calling the 'upper frame', that is, with a high stance. We all trained basic *zenkutsu-dachi* front-stance in a 'low frame' because, he said, 'this was good for developing strong leg muscles'.

Usually, in basic form, the front kick is deployed from the back leg, although in competition many will develop it from the leading foot because it is quicker. In this session kicking from the leading foot 'was' the basic method. We skipped the back leg up to the front and then lifted the knee high to deliver *maegeri*. But rather than the usual 'snap in and out' commonly taught in Shotokan the Old Man's technique was more like a cross between a snap kick and a stomp kick. It penetrated and trod onto the opponent, sometimes into the hip line to cut the attacker short from advancing. On the punchbag he used his big toe and then demonstrated the same on the concrete pillar. Then where it should strike on an attacker.

If you were old and couldn't lift your knee high then you kicked into the hock of someones ankle or calf muscle. Other targets for the big toe include a point in the hollow just above the knee on the outside of the leg. A third point can be found by placing your small finger on this hollow and stretching your hand wide until your thumb rests naturally upon another target high on the outside of the thigh, the infamous 'dead leg' point of school playground days. Here a toe kick or simple knee attack was enough to bring a taller opponent down in line with your new *age-uke* styled punch. But of course it wasn't new, it was old.

The lesson ended far too soon.

Afterwards I loitered with a small group of seniors in the hope of gleaming more from the Old Man. He seemed to be lecturing one of the younger sensei about 'mysticism' in karate. Lecturing but in a relaxed and informal way. The way a senior *sempai* might coach a junior; guiding but not demanding.

For his part the younger sensei appeared to entertain the Old Man. He wasn't disrespectful in any way but, as much of the university crowd appeared too, he simply smiled and nodded along politely. A German who had been training in the class grinned at me standing on the sidelines trying desperately to pick out the words being used.

"He is telling sensei to become more spiritual. That in karate it is important to understand '*ki*' and 'supernatural things'. He says that karate is loosing these things and that sensei should start to explore them so that they are not lost forever, but kept alive for the next generation" I nodded in agreement. The sensei grinned and shook his head and the Old Man looked at me.

"Do you think he is right?" The German student now asked with an almost mocking tone in his voice.

"Hai." I replied.

It struck me that karate, or at least Shotokan, was missing these things. The other group I'd arrived in Japan with had spoken of controlling time and space, hypnosis, even gamma rays and infra-red. The logic being that these things are in the atmosphere and all around us and that through increased sensitivity one could experience their existence. In theory it made sense to me.

In the Bujinkan dojo Hatsumi sensei taught how to use psychology and subtle body movements to distract, disorientate and manipulate an opponent. Not just opponents but people in general. I'd also heard tales of Ucshiba Morihei, the founder of Aikido, a martial art that empowers practitioners to turn an aggressor's attack upon themselves into a safe takedown.

Ueshiba spoke of seeing 'rays of light' moving before an opponent's physical attack even took place. He felt it was their intent. There are countless stories in the martial arts of people demonstrating such abilities or speaking in such terms. For many it is part of what attracts them to learning the martial arts in the first place. What the Old Man was discussing now did not seem so far-fetched or unreasonable.

Hirokazu Kanazawa used to strike a stack of wooden planks and direct the focus of his force into just the middle one. Only this plank would break and the others on each side remained un-harmed. It's a more widely known party-trick these days but Kanazawa's explanation was that "The fist fills a space in time already occupied by the mind." As far as I'm aware that is about the most mystical thing ever described by an exponent of Shotokan.

For me the expense of relocating into the heart of Tokyo for a week was well worth the opportunity of meeting this Old Man for just one morning. The lesson at the dojo had ended but for me Fate had one more surprise up her sleeve. It turned out the Old Man and I were to share the first part of our journey home. His English was limited but it didn't seem to matter because he continued to discuss and demonstrate more techniques and the language of martial arts is universal.

We walked into a small park and paused. Turning he encouraged me to grab the lapel of his jacket. "Take!" As I did he cupped my fist in his palm and buried the tip of his thumb into a pressure-point on the top of my hand. The pain was electrifying as he effortlessly turned my hand over into a wrist lock which caused me to drop to one knee flapping in submission. He let go and laughed still holding his hand in the half 'prayer like' position the technique had ended in. He nodded and smiled bringing both palms together into a sort of prayer gesture. "*Gassho*! hmm?" Then just one hand to emphasise a point "Te." I massaged my wrist and his open hand became a fist "Karate. Hai? Karate, Te. Hai?

There was that word again 'Te', an ancient martial art that had ceased to be practiced by the eighteen hundreds. Yet here, in this quiet little park the Old Man hinted that the techniques he was now showing me were part of that old and once secret martial art. They were, as he described them, some of the techniques Funakoshi used to teach him during those formative years when he first introduced Okinawan martial arts to the mainland.

"Take!" Prompting me eagerly he now proffered a wrist to grab. Glancing around I seized about his wrist with a firm grip. Within an instant it felt like a bolt of electricity had shot up my arm and I was down on one knee with my wrist caught in his powerful grasp once more. No sooner had the pain come on it was gone. I looked up, confused and excited all at once. The Old Man was powerfully built for his age. He had what I called an 'awkward strength' that elder men like my grandfather used to possess. But it wasn't muscular power he used to apply the techniques. In the class earlier it was clear he could hit hard, but now his movements were achieved with a certain softness. They appeared almost effortless.

Seeing I was ok he nodded and I started to stand again. My wrist still trapped in his grip. As I made it to my feet he drew attention to the hold and subtly applied a little pressure which caused the pain to come back in a flash. He chuckled as I winced and did it again. On and off like a switch. The feeling reminded me of the stories Funakoshi recounted about his teacher who, it was said, had a vice like grip that felt like the bones in your wrists were being crushed.

The grip the Old Man had taken upon me was much the same as how you would hold a sword or any weapon in the Japanese martial arts. The smallest finger of course was tightly sealed but the index finger, the most important, was not tight. It was relaxed. When a wrist is grabbed in this way the underside of the largest knuckle of the index finger, as well as the thumb and tips of the smaller fingers, all naturally rest upon a series of pressure-points that can be manipulated to cause pain. As no muscles can be developed around the wrist it doesn't matter what size an opponent is because the points will always be easily manipulated. This is what causes the 'crushing' feeling or the 'vice-like' grip attributed to the masters of old.

With this method you can control an opponent. If pressure is applied correctly to the inside of the opponent's wrist the pain will cause them to move in the opposite direction to escape. Press upon the outside and the reverse is true. Bring pressure against the underside of the wrist, where the veins are easily seen, and a person is likely to rise onto their toes while pressing upon the top of the wrist will cause them to sink. By taking the hand, or rather wrists, you can direct an opponent's movements by simply moving through the basic 'block' or '*uke*' techniques of all karate styles. Directional gripping.

Funakoshi used to say 'grasp a strong man loosely and a weak man firmly.'

The Old Man was undeniably strong but he didn't rely upon this muscular strength. Instead his stability and rootedness came from much lower down in his *hara*, which was big and round. When he applied his grips they weren't 'full on' until the moment he wanted them to be, and then, because of his awareness of the body's anatomical weak-spots, the grip was intense.

Releasing my wrist he stepped back and nodded.

"Punch!" He took a relaxed posture and tapped his chest. He nodded again. I felt a little un-easy. Not because of past memories of teachers urging me to hit them, I did not feel threatened here at all, I felt uneasy because of how it might look if someone were to walk into the park. Me a young westerner trying to punch the Old Man. But this was a lesson and he was telling me to hit him.

I didn't adopt much of a stance I just lifted my *kamae*, fighting posture, and rushed forward with a punch. His own posture seemed hopelessly defenceless. He just stood with hands relaxed by his sides. But in the moment I was about to hit he was gone. He'd moved just enough to slip my punch and at the same time struck a knuckle jab into my ribs and anchored a foot to jar my lead leg. Like the judo children in Ayase his jab became a grab upon my clothing and he tugged me forward into a throw.

My palms grated into the gravel path and he stood behind me as if nothing had happened. He tapped his chest again.

"Attack." Dusting myself off I tried once more. This time he slipped inside my punch. An open hand shot to my throat while his other seized about my wrist and had me squirming again as the pressure of his grip came on. With a simple turn of his footwork I came tumbling off balance once more. Then he clenched both fists and clashed them into each other, demonstrating in his charades-type way to explain.

"Only strongest win." I attacked again and he stepped aside at the final moment and tripped my back foot away.

"No block." He crashed his fists together again to emphasise the point of strongest wins. He was showing me, or rather teaching me, in a very experiential way that non-confrontation was the best way to secure victory. When force meets force only the strongest will win; and both are likely to be injured.

In the regular classes of the dojo I would often come home with bruised forearms from all the hard blocking techniques you had to perform in fixed *kumite* drills. An attacker would strongly enter and naturally you would want to get out of the way but Shotokan seemed to dictate that you must hold your ground and block hard. Here the Old Man was saying not to block. That karate blocks are not really blocks at all but strikes. Each time I'd attacked him he did not get in the way or try to stop my movement he simply avoided a clash and entered in with his counter.

He looked over my shoulder and helped me up off the ground once more. An elderly couple had entered the park and so we headed off. Walking on he tried to explain in greater depth but language proved too difficult. I captured words, Okinawa, *Shuri*, *bujutsu*. But the details remained clouded. We made our way to the train station and that is where we parted company.

I never saw the Old Man again. It was an enlightening morning by all accounts and in the years that followed I cannot recall the number of times I've kicked myself for not being able to communicate more clearly with him. To ask him more. To thank him for setting me upon the path he did. But sometimes that's how it goes.

The next morning I woke from a curious dream. I was walking up a mountain path with a donkey in tow. The sun-baked dusty path went up and up high above a jungle forest canopy down below. Eventually I arrived at a steel door. On the other side was a concrete bunker, like a large pill-box structure from WWII and seated around a table were three of my brothers, all in military uniforms. Then, from another door, my last brother entered. He handed me a rolled parchment scroll and as I took it from him I woke up.

It wasn't so much the content of the dream that caused me to write it down in my journal but more the feeling that accompanied it upon waking. From the tips of my toes all the way to the crown of my head my whole body was vibrating with an intense tingling sensation. It was not too dissimilar to 'pins and needles', perhaps more like a mild electric shock, but nowhere near as uncomfortable or debilitating. I laid in bed and bathed in this new sensation. It lasted about fifteen minutes before slowly ebbing away. On some level it lingered for the day because I felt like I'd had a 'power up' and could accomplish anything or take on anyone. I was vibrant and full of energy.

My time in Japan was naturally drawing to a close. In Tokyo the famous Sarin Subway Incident had brought disruption and death through a series of domestic terrorism attacks. In late June a man claiming to be a member of the group hijacked an All Japan Airways plane with 350 passengers onboard. Initial reports suggested he had explosives. The event dominated the twenty-four hour news channels and back at the apartment Sasha and I watched as a small corner of the screen was dedicated to a live feed of the cockpit as the plane sat on a runway.

We couldn't understand the logic of it. Had a hijacker been so inclined to make a very strong impression he could have executed a crew member on live national television. But now it wasn't certain if he had explosives at all, but perhaps a gun?

A few days later and it was still going on. After training one evening I asked Masakazu "don't you have a special forces team that will storm the plane?"

"Oh no! That would be VERY bad."
"Really? Why bad?"
"If the military go in they will shoot him."
"But he is threatening to kill 350 people!"
"Yes but killing him will make us as bad as him."
"So what will happen?"
"He is probably getting very tired now. He is alone. They might send the riot police."

And that is what they did. To be fair the Tokyo Riot Police is a strong force to be reckoned with and it seems storming a hijacked plane falls within their mandate. It turned out that the hijacker was armed with a sharpened screwdriver.

The whole thing started to make me wonder if Japan really understood how dangerous the rest of the world could be. I found myself worrying and at the same time becoming agitated by the lack of valiant spirit that once dominated Japanese culture. Where was this warrior spirit now? How could one individual hold up a plane full of passengers with a just a screwdriver without being taken down by someone?

Of course my concerns were ridiculous. Japan had suffered a great deal at the end of the Second World War and, as a nation, were well aware of how dangerous the rest of the world could be.

Having emerged from centuries of internal warfare, where the egos of warlords clashed with each other in the pursuit of power, Japan had truly evolved into a peaceful nation. The martial arts still played a key role in the upbringing of school children and much of the culture and work ethos of the industrial boom following the war had spurned the Japanese to forge a strong economy. Business became war and they excelled at it. In the process it seemed the general psyche of the population had also evolved to realise the enlightened principle that the Old Man had taught me in the park. A strategy that was at the heart of Funakoshi's teachings and the origins of Okinawan martial arts themselves; the way of non-confrontation.

9
Whispers from the past
"Unlocking the 'Te' in Funakoshi's karate."

'*...I recall, when I was a child, hearing my elders speak of both "Okinawa-te" and "karate". I began then to think of Okinawa-te as an indigenous Okinawan fighting art and of karate as a Chinese form of boxing. In any case, I perceived a clear distinction between the two.*'

Gichin Funakoshi
MY WAY OF LIFE

The following year, back in England, I took to studying everything I could find on Funakoshi. I re-read his books inside and out and, whenever possible, sourced collectable first editions for comparison. I searched for hints of the master's original art in writings and film.

Pictorially there were big differences between the stances and postures used in his early work *Rentan Goshin Toudi Jutsu*, and those in a later re-write titled *Karate-Dō Kyōhan*, 'Way of Karate - The Master Text'. Although much of the written content remained the same the images used in the works depicted a vastly different stye than that which first arrived from Okinawa in the 1920's. After the master's death the images of the books replaced the old with the new favouring the more fashionable dynamic techniques of Shotokan today. Such techniques were created with fitness and competition in mind and they held limited 'street value' as a fighting art. In turn this move has led to stylists of other karate schools to doubt the effectiveness of Funakoshi's martial ability. The more I searched the more I came to feel that such criticisms might be unfounded.

Funakoshi's other works included *Karate Dō Nyumon*, 'The Introductory Text', and his autobiography '*My Way of Life*'. In these he recorded memories of his early life on Okinawa and the oral teachings of his teachers in martial arts. People like Asato and Itosu. With new eyes I found his words littered with hints of the Te he learnt in his formative years from his main teacher Asato.

Yasatsune Asato was a senior member of the ruling 'Shizoku' class and held the title *Tonochi*, the second highest rank below the King himself. His family presided over the village of Asato which is now part of the modern day Okinawan capital of Naha.

Funakoshi was also born Shizoku. His father was a low ranking official who worked at the Royal Palace and was skilled in classical dance, singing and *bojutsu* stick-fighting. Funakoshi's introduction to Asato no doubt was influenced via his father's connections. In fact, Funakoshi's grandfather had also served within the palace where he taught Chinese Classics to the kings concubines.

Under Asato, the young Funakoshi learnt the fundamentals of Te. Early photo's of Funakoshi leading a group of Okinawan martial artists on the mainland show them posed with various kobudo weapons, suggesting that at the least he had a grasp of the fundamentals of weaponry too. Later Funakoshi trained with Itosu in the Chinese kung-fu and Te hybrid called *Tode*, that would ultimately become karate proper. Then, from time to time upon the introduction of these two masters, Funakoshi also received instruction from the kings chief bodyguard Sokon Matsumura.

Funakoshi wrote very little about Te as a separate art from karate. Perhaps in his time the boundary between the two disciplines had already become hazy because frequently he described Te as karate and karate as Te. I even started to wonder if there was a difference between the two myself. It was only the lessons from the Old Man in the park that made me persevere in my search and then I found a spattering of historical references that made a clear distinction between Te and Karate.

The earliest record of the term karate appears in an 18th century document titled the Oshima Hikki, the 'incident' at Oshima.

Authored by a resident monk the Oshima Hikki records the unfortunate ship wrecking of a Ryukyuan vessel on the shores of Oshima Island. At one point a conversation about martial arts came up and the ship's Captain recounted to the monk his impressions of a situation which he'd witnessed in Shuri the previous year.

At the time Okinawa was the seat of power of the Ryukyu Kingdom, a semi-independent tributary state to China that flourished through maritime trade. This tributary status meant that every time a new king was crowned China would acknowledge proceedings by dispatching a fully laden 'Crown Ship' to Shuri bearing gifts and documents officiating the new kings authority. These were big affairs involving hundreds of envoys and the fleet would swell with merchant ships keen to take advantage of the protection offered from the escorting Imperial vessels as they crossed the East China Sea.

The investiture missions would arrive in Okinawa and usually stay for several months before making the return journey to China. The 1756 mission, dispatched to celebrate the crowning of king Shō Boku was led by a senior envoy known as Kwan Ku. The original ship apparently ran aground on Kume Island to the west of Okinawa and the surviving crew returned to China where a new ship was outfitted and dispatched, arriving in Okinawa in winter and staying for seven months.

Whilst there it seems a series of disturbances broke out between the Chinese merchants and the Okinawans as they tried to forcefully unload their wares. The authorities were called and Kwan Ku appears to have taken a part in either settling the trouble or the edifications that followed. In either case the Captain of the Oshima Hikki recounts his impressions of Kwan Ku using his legs in the fashion of a crab's claws to fell larger opponents.

The Chinese official's fighting style clearly left a lasting impression with the martial artists of the day. Not only did a young apprentice cartographer named Kanga Sakugawa return to China to learn Kwan Ku's method but a number of karate kata today still bear his name under various adaptations; *Kwanku*, *Kushanku*, *Kanku*. As kata can be said to be an expression of thought patterns then it is clear Kwan Ku's skill lived on in memory within the Okinawan martial arts community.

When Kwan Ku set off to China, Shō Boku awarded him fifty thousand ounces of silver as compensation for the original goods lost in transit but when this gift was presented to the Emperor in China he flew into a rage. Ryukyu was too small a nation to afford such a generous gift and he insisted "It must be returned". When he heard about the trouble in Naha he had those directly involved either executed, beaten or decommissioned in rank. Only Kwan Ku seems to have avoided being rebuked. Who knows, perhaps that was in part Sakugawa's role to express the Kings gratitude for his services?

A few years later Sakugawa returned to Okinawa where he was awarded the nick name 'Tode' Sakugawa on the count of his expertise in Chinese martial arts. He became a senior security advisor to the king, a role his own disciple Matsumura, would later inherit.

How does all this prove that an art called Te existed in Okinawa? That Sakugawa gained the nickname '*Tode*', 'Chinese Hand', strongly suggests that another fighting art more indigenous to the islands already existed. Otherwise why wasn't he simply known as Te Sakugawa?

In The Essence of Okinawan Karate-Dō Shoshin Nagamine makes the same point and also highlights another example of Te which outdates the use of the term *Tode* by nearly a hundred years.

'That there was a difference between Te and the Chinese-style self-defence can be illustrated in both poetry and history.

A poem by the eminent Okinawan scholar Nage Uekata, whose birth in 1663 antedates by ninety-eight years the first recorded performance of Chinese-style self-defence on Okinawa, mentions Te in a very significant context. The poem reads in part:

*"No matter how you excel in the art of te,
and in your scholastic endeavours,
nothing is more important than your behaviour
and your humanity as observed in daily life."'*

There were other hints of this elusive art called Te too. In 1882 Sokon Matsumura, the kings bodyguard, wrote down his advice on the virtues of academic and martial arts study to his senior student. In it he categorises fighting arts as belonging to three groups, those of Court instructors, nominal styles and true fighting arts.

"The court instructors' styles are practised in a very unusual way; movements are never the same, formless and light, becoming, like women, more dance-like as the proponents mature."

The observation of this dance-like quality of movement is significant. When the Japanese invaded Okinawa in 1609 they imposed greater restrictions upon the shizoku class carrying personal arms and studying military arts. The techniques of Te, which had evolved from ancient times and were honed in a period of civil war went underground. Ultimately they were codified and concealed within the soft, meditative movements of a new dance genre that emerged within the palace from 1719. This distinctive operatic style, called *kumiodori*, was performed exclusively by the sons of the aristocracy. People like Funakoshi's father.

In these performances they dressed in traditional women's costume to emphasise the 'feminine' yielding nature of the Te techniques hidden within. Their songs and stories re-told the glory of the Ryukyu Kingdom's rise to power and the lessons of its tribulations along the way.

Discrete props such as parasols, paper fans and willow sprigs replaced swords, bows and glaives, the weapons of Te. The movements, though slow like Tai-chi, mirrored the techniques of the fighting art with absolute perfection. The oldest dances, the 'Women's Dances' *Onna-Odori*, effectively became a catalogue of Te's repertoire and layered within their movements existed the wisdom of longevity and exercises for the nourishment of intrinsic energy. *Ki*.

Collectively the dances were called '*Te-odori*', 'dance hand', and in later generations the movements became more expressive and reflected the trends of more fashionable fighting techniques such as karate and kobudo, it's non-bladed weapon based sister art. This argument of classical dance linking to Te is strengthened by the observation that most folk dances on Okinawa today are reminiscent of karate movements with obvious punches, leg stomps and grimacing faces, whereas the older 'court' dances remain sedate and reflective of an older, more refined, court culture.

Matsumura most likely experienced great frustration with Te and significant prejudice from members of the ruling aristocracy of the time. Despite gaining the titled rank of Bushi, or 'knight' and serving as the kings chief bodyguard, he was not born of nobility and therefore would have been excluded from learning the art of Te in any great depth. As a bodyguard he naturally would have wanted control of how the King reacted in threatening situations and on occasion he instructed him in his own pugilistic method that focussed on fast knockdown strikes. But the official role of teaching martial arts to the king belonged to one family alone. The Motobu's.

The Motobu's were connected to the crown by blood and carried the title of *Udun*. For nearly four hundred years a Motobu had instructed the King and Heir Apparent in the methods of their art. It became a closely guarded secret handed down from father to eldest son for over eleven generations. It taught not only martial arts but psychology and strategy too.

Matsumura, and indeed many of the officials of the palace who were versed in martial arts were ultimately 'hired muscle'. They were positioned in such a way as to form a concealed fighting force should the occasion ever require it. But could a Head of State ever be truly trusting of his close security? Would it not be prudent to hold something back in case of betrayal? For this reason, and others, it was deemed that the Palace 'Hand' method remained secret so that in the most extreme of events, a *coup d'ètat* for example, the King had his own means of escaping danger.

In contrast to Matsumura's preference for fast, hard hitting strikes and the teachings of Itosu which favoured grounded physical power it seems that Te incorporated lighter techniques such as jumping, kicking and even somersaults. The last Grandmaster of Motobu Udundi, perhaps the purest Te style to exist today, was Seikichi Uehara. He lived to a hundred and passed away in 2004. Uehara's early training included such unusual practices such as jumping from graves and climbing walls whilst punching and kicking.

Another Te expert in Matsumura's time was Bushi Tachimura. In Mark Bishop's '*Okinawan Karate, Teachers, Styles & Secret Techniques*' he includes the following story recounted to him by his teacher Higa Seitoku:

'Takemura and the elderly master Sokon Matsumura had been good friends. Once whilst they were drinking together in the garden of a country estate at Shikina near Shuri, Takemura teased Matsumura by saying he was too old to do anything. A friendly match thus being provoked, Takemura started to rise from his cross-legged sitting position and had just raised one knee when Matsumura attempted to scoop his leg, but instead of being thrown, Takemura floated gracefully through the air, did a perfect back somersault and landed gently on a small stone bridge over a carp pond.

Matsumura was so taken aback at seeing this exhibition of levitation that he ran into his house and failed to reappear for the rest of the evening.'

No doubt the story, like many recounted on Okinawa about past masters, has been embellished over the years. Or perhaps not. What can be gleamed with certainty is that again a description of Te highlights the importance of suppleness and the use of jumping and acrobatics.

I began to wonder what, if any, of the former Te of Asato had been handed down into modern Shotokan via Funakoshi.

In essence I came to feel that Te, as a martial art, was largely principle based whereas techniques in karate are more physical and straight forward. The difference being that the later were more reflective of linear thought patterns and the former an expression of lateral thinking. Karate was an 'external' martial art and Te was 'internal'.

From Matsumura's perspective Te appeared fluid and dance-like, formless and light with no two movements ever being the same. In contrast, his karate style was direct and forceful, dynamic and no-nonsense. It could be taught to a group in militant fashion. Te was the opposite. No pre-arrangement. No fixed ideas and no specific planned response, because you can never truly plan for every possibility. Instead it taught to calm the mind, nurture inner balance and heighten sensitivity. In a zen-like way Te enabled an individual to live 'in the moment' and not worry about the future; for in truth the future can only be crafted in the present anyway.

Matsumura once described Te as a 'game of psychology and tactics' demonstrating that the expressions of Te he'd encountered showed it to be a principle centric art. But what does that mean?

Principles are eternal snippets of wisdom that embody the philosophic intentions of a master's technique. Whereas physical techniques can become altered and changed by others over time, principles remain the same. Funakoshi penned twenty such principles as a lasting testament for those dedicated students of karate seeking truth.

Known as the *Niju-Kun* they embody a great deal of the wisdom that Funakoshi perhaps gleamed from his teacher Asato. In many ways I came to feel that whereas the techniques of Shotokan, later enhanced or altered by Funakoshi's son Gigo, would become the vehicle by which some of Itosu's and Matsumura's martial art knowledge was preserved into the future, the *Niju-Kun* preserved the lessons of Asato's style.

At the time of compiling the Niju-kun Funakoshi felt socially obligated to disguise not only the arts Chinese influences but also any aspects of Ryukyuan culture as being distinct from Japan. Being born at a time when the Ryukyu Kingdom was officially being annexed into the modern Japanese Empire he witnessed great social reforms and a period of 'naturalisation'. So effective were the Japanese at wiping out traces of Okinawa's former existence as an independent nation that even today it is not uncommon for younger generations of mainlanders to reference Okinawans in a somewhat ignorant and derogatory way. "They are provincial farmers" was quoted to me more than once during my stay in Japan.

For these reasons, when Funakoshi writes the word karate he is usually speaking of both Te and the later hybrid of Te and Chinese kung-fu which became 'karate'. Searching for the clues of Te's existence became challenging but there were principles of Te hidden within the twenty points and old photo's in his books before the big change.

Article 17 states: '*Kamae wa shoshinsha ni ato wa shizentai*' 'Stances are for beginners, then use natural posture'. This is very reflective of Te's 'non confrontational' approach to strategy. When two fighters meet it is common in karate to adopt postures and stances that reflect your fighting style. In boxing they have 'guard' positions. Whether in fencing or empty-hand combat each 'attitude' or 'posture' reveals to the opponent something of your strategy. By adopting no-stance, or rather a natural one, all options are open and you give no clues to the enemy. Te has no fixed *kamae*.

When I faced the Old Man in the park his stance appeared hopeless until the very last moment my attack was about to strike. When I rode the train with Mr Sawada he'd demonstrated the same 'relaxed' natural ready stance.

Many of the original photo's used in Funakoshi's early books showed the use of a stance called "T-stance" which is strikingly similar to the posture used in classical *Kumiodori* dance performances. Although modern translations depict the more powerful looking front-stance the footnotes still reference when T-stance would have originally been used.

But if there is any doubt about whether Asato's 'Te' is concealed within Funakoshi's Niju-kun then it is clearly found within item 15. '*Hito no teashi wo ken to omou*', 'Think of a persons' hands and feet as swords'. This is the opposite of Itosu's advice of 'making the body hard enough to repel all strikes'.

All too often in Shotokan, and karate dojo's in general, it has become 'acceptable' to allow an opponent to land a blow to hardened parts of the body so as to gain an advantage or create openings in their defence. This is born from sporting competition, but in real combat, where knives or concealed 'street weapons' are often used, it is dangerous to allow any contact. By thinking of your opponent's hands and feet as swords you will move in a totally different way. You will avoid all contact from them.

Over the next few years I would find myself working door security to a number of troubled venues throughout West London. From these experiences I came to realise two simple assumptions about karate training with regards to self-defence. First, if you are unfortunate to find yourself in a fight, assume you'll be outnumbered because gone are the days of gentlemen taking off their jackets and 'stepping outside' for a one to one. Secondly, your attackers will most likely be armed to increase their chance of victory.

Few people realise until after the event but in more cases than not the aggressor either had a knife or used some other item, be it a glass, bottle or ashtray. Outnumbered and armed.

It is from this understanding that those interested in developing their karate for self-defence purposes should really start analysing *kata bunkai*. And if you think street brawls two hundred years ago in Okinawa were calmer affairs than those seen outside clubs and bars today think again. Hatchets, blades, knuckle dusters and more were used with just as much frequency then as now. Even in Funakoshi's time deaths were common.

The difference perhaps is that Funakoshi moved within the circles of the upper-class and for this reason his martial arts took on a lot of the ethical values of true '*bu*' training and the preservation of peace.

From all the hints and snippets I'd amassed from Funakoshi's writings and teachings, as well as the lessons taught by the Old Man, I reasoned that in Te I was looking for a fluid and non-power-based martial art. I reasoned that the techniques would be fast and used natural postures and weaponry too. It would be non-confrontational in it's application and presumably more 'principle' based in order to apply to a wider range of situations. Logically then, Te would be an art with few techniques, but those few techniques could be applied in a limitless number of ways.

A paradigm shift in my thinking was occurring. My karate world was being turned upside down and I began looking at things in a different way. If the *Nijukun* contained hints of Funakoshi's 'Te' training did something of modern Shotokan too? It was time to speak to a man who had experience of Te first hand.

10
Te Time

"In the shadow of the mountains
our dojo had no walls"

"Breakfast has to be earned." Winter. France. After several years of tracking down Mark Bishop I'd arrived at his rustic farmhouse close to the Midi-Pyrenees. Actually we'd arrived the evening before and unable to get the boiler working had had a cold night and even colder morning. Jack Frost had breathed upon the single-pane windows to my stone-walled bedroom and as I opened the storm shutters Mark was stretching on the veranda outside. The house rule, the only one really, was that breakfast cost a brief stretch and short jog; a healthy rule by any standards and one that never gave me cause to grumble.

I'd come to live with Mark and train in his eclectic approach to Te which focusses extensively on weaponry and pressure-point manipulation. Years earlier, when I first returned from Japan, I'd continued my shiatsu training under Mark enjoying he's liberated and intuitive method which reflected the shiatsu of yesteryear. In Tokyo shiatsu had long become clinical and mainstream with an application similar to the way osteopathy and physiotherapy is practised here in the West. In contrast Mark's shiatsu was fluid, best practised at floor level and deeply powerful. He'd learnt it whilst living in Okinawa between the late seventies to early nineties as well as karate, kobudo and Te from various sources. He had spent over fifteen years on the islands teaching English and starting a family. During his spare time he made a point of visiting many of the ageing karate masters of that period, cataloguing their stylistic differences and the official lineages of their respective styles. All of this was compiled into his hugely successful book *'Okinawan Karate, Teachers, Styles & Secret Techniques'*.

In exchange for my board and tuition, I'd agreed to help him finalise and prepare two more manuscripts for publication which he'd written in the years since *Okinawan Karate* came out. The first of these was a sequel of sorts titled *'Okinawan Weaponry'* and the second, *'Zen Odyssey'*, was a personal account of his time on the islands and the situations he encountered.

Whereas *Okinawan Karate* subtly led the reader from what was considered the most rudimentary to the more refined of karate styles, concluding with a chapter introducing the Te styles, *Okinawan Weaponry* delved deeper into the history of kobudo and the preservation of Te from the 7th century onwards.

In many dojo's today weaponry practise is usually reserved for 'advanced' trainees, which often leads to the misconception that training with weapons is equal to 'advanced' training; which then leads to the misbelief that empty-hand fighting comes before weaponry; when in actual fact the opposite is true.

Man, being the weakest of the apes, has always needed to exercise intelligence over braun in order to survive against wild beasts and adversaries. Thus our earliest ancestors, even in stone age times, used stick, rock and bone to first strengthen their defence and then improve hunting ability. Even today the training of frontline troops focusses predominantly on use of firearms and very little on hand to hand combat. Five hundred years ago things weren't much different. Empty hand fighting is always a last resort and certainly the least desired. In Te the relationship between weaponry use and empty-hand technique is intricately linked, so much so that it is often said one trained only in the empty-hand aspects of the Te can readily adapt their skill to any object or weapon close to hand.

On a practical level, continued training with classical weapons such as the bow, sword and spear, help to refine fundamental empty-hand techniques such as punches, strikes and grabs because they amplify minor faults. Like using a cue in the game of Snooker or Pool, poor technique in gripping and preparing a shot will result in poor play upon the ball at the end of the four foot stick. The same is true of weaponry in martial arts. So using a spear for example can amplify faults in gripping and punching technique too.

For several years Mark had not taught anyone and it took some coaxing to gain the opportunity to live and train with him. Helping to edit and prepare the manuscripts was a fair exchange and provided a rare chance to study under a teacher who really does 'live his art'.

My morning workouts began with stretching and breathing exercises in order to open the lungs, release the fatigue of sleep and nourish the blood. This was followed by a brisk jog in the style peculiar to Te with shoulders dropped, heels lifted and breathing from the *hara*. This 'trotting' type technique is what enabled the Shuri Guard to mobilise along the cobbled roads of Okinawa in order to head off invading forces or *Wako* pirate raids during turbulent times. The technique enables one to traverse distances at a reasonable pace and arrive at a destination fresh and alert for combat. Modern soldiers in the British Forces use a similar method today which they call TAB'ing, an acronym for 'Tactical Advance to Battle'.

Having never been fond of jogging or running before I surprisingly came to enjoy this morning routine and soon extended my route along the country lanes and through the surrounding hills about the farm. Years later I would discover that this method of jogging, like so many of the advanced techniques of Te, could also be traced to the ancient shamanistic practises of Okinawa's female priestess caste known as *noro*.

Not only were these jogs good for clearing the mind but waking exercise, even if only for a short time, works wonders for the digestive system and prevents a sluggish fatigue setting in during the afternoon.

After a jog came breakfast; it had after all now been earned. The day ahead would then follow a loose structure, never regimented or strict but always purposeful, wholesome and balanced. For example a typical day might continue with manual work about the property. The farmhouse was over one hundred years old and its solid walls had been constructed with large rounded rocks shaped during the last glacial period, a time when Northern Europe was compounded under miles of ice and tundra. Now the farmland around was arid and wild having long been abandoned years ago.

Before the heat of midday we'd either clear brush and bramble, gather firewood, dig new irrigation trenches or collect rocks to repair broken walls. Slowly but surely the two bedroom house with its central hearth room and kitchen gained an additional bathroom and several bedrooms reclaimed from derelict neglect, while the surrounding land and outbuildings equally benefited from a new breath of life too.

Everything was related to training, breathing and living. For example the curved bladed mattock-hoe was used with footwork that picked and danced through fallen nettle and vine and replaced the curve bladed *naginata*. The practise was reminiscent of battlefield fighting where one had to be ever mobile in order to avoid cuts to the legs from neighbouring comrades and flailing enemy weapons. Shovel and spade made for *hara* development, raking the ground improved handling of the spear and chopping with the two-handed axe attuned the breathing and timing necessary for sword work.

By late morning we'd rest and enjoy a freshly ground coffee. It was peaceful on the farm, and when the sun was out it blessed the tiled veranda making it a perfect place to sit, ponder a thought and share a memory. Then a little more work and a second training session followed in the late afternoon. These sessions always had a certain format commencing with partner stretches to open the body followed by footwork, weaponry and *kumite*. This *kumite* was free-form and varied. It included basic strikes and avoidance, weapon versus weapon and then empty hand versus weapon.

Most of the training stayed on a *kumite* level and in this way lessons were learnt through direct experience. In the shadow of the mountains our dojo had no walls and our *kumite* had no restrictions. If you didn't move fast enough you got hit, if you gripped your weapon poorly your knuckles were smashed by incoming strikes with the staff, *tonfa* or *bokken*. The rain served to improve Te footwork and taught not to lunge forward through risk of losing balance or sliding in the mud. In the early days defeat followed defeat fuelling flames of anger and frustration until inevitably I'd rush forward with furious determination to land a blow but ever find myself hurled into air or tumbling down a slope into the field below. Yet through all this not once did my teacher loose his cool; my brashness was always met with patience and composure.

In the evenings, after a hot meal and shower, we would sit down to work upon the books late into the night. These sessions took place before the warming crackle and glow of an open fire with discussions and occasional impromptu demonstrations of technique to help elicit a key point. The books, for the most part, were already written and the work mainly consisted of compiling and structuring the content coherently. A wealth of information came out through conversation and recollection, not all of which could fit upon the pages, and so for several months my training was enriched not only through the study of Te technique but also through oral tradition and the passing down of wisdom.

✻

"Street fighters attack with the head, teeth and knees so the primary defence in Te is to protect the eyes, ears and groin …"

A cold November morning I found myself down on one knee recovering from the intense pressure point massage my face had just received as a result of Mark's swift defence. Moments earlier I'd swung a six-foot stick at his head only to have him deftly slip inside the arc, snare my wrist with one hand and thrust his thumb and fingers painfully into my face with the other. In the blink of an eye he'd rolled the crude weapon from my grip, jabbed its short end into a pressure point in my ribs and tripped me to the frost hardened ground.

Now pinned by his boot treading on my outstretched hand he explained the more practical side of Te's approach to self-defence.

"When an attack comes just enter and expand."

By expansion he meant rising to your toes reaching out and striking the face with your fingertips. Eyes are primary targets, then there are points below the eyes, the temples, in the cheeks and under the jaw. More points can be found in the hollow behind the ears, the throat and neck. As a shiatsu practitioner I can think of at least twenty-six locations off the top of my head. Which means with the four fingers and thumb of an open hand you've got a high chance of striking several pressure-points at once.

This was how our private training took place and the lessons were directly ingrained through application to points or '*tsubo*'. After all, we learn more from pain and the avoidance of it than we do from pleasure.

Today a lot of karate-ka train in pressure-point fighting. Essentially a pressure point is a location where the nervous or circulatory system can be stimulated through striking, grabbing, pressing or squeezing. 'Vital points' are usually junctures where these systems cross over each other and double the effect of a strike. In Te, just like shiatsu, we don't follow 'fixed' points like an exponent of *Dim-Mak* or *Kyusho Jutsu* might do, and there are no 'set-up' techniques either like "press point 'B' to make point 'X' more vulnerable", the body just doesn't work that way and neither does real fighting.

In shiatsu you learn that points are more painful and tender when there is tension surrounding them. The aim of shiatsu is to release this tension in order to restore health, but in karate the aim will be to cause injury. Yet in Te, at an advanced level, the aim is again to release tension. In this way training becomes like a form of bodywork similar to shiatsu in itself.

The key then is not to see the body as a map of intricate switches that can be flicked on and off at will but rather a living entity that responds to external stimuli. In Te we enter into an attackers space and reach out to strike or seize whatever points happen to be there, and if the opponent tries to recoil or continue with a second attack their movement will always reveal more targets in the process.

"Now you try." Dusting myself off, Mark positioned himself ahead of me with the stick. Behind him the snow-capped crests of the Pyrenees formed an awesome backdrop to what had become our 'outdoor' dojo, a small patch of land overlooking the farm and sheltered from the road by a hedgerow.

The speed of his first strike took me a little by surprise and rather than move lightly, like I'd been taught, I sunk low and heard the weapon 'whomp' overhead. Quick on the return he spun around just as I dived forward into a roll to avoid the obvious strike to my exposed back. Turning in the roll and springing back to my feet all I could really do was propel myself forward with a hop-kick and double strike as his third swing circled to the side of my head again.

It was close but my leap got me just inside. Driving a palm strike to the nose my splayed fingers squeezed upon his temples while I trapped the weapon under my other arm. I tried to manipulate an elbow point through his thick jacket and followed with a knee attack to a point on his thigh. A tangled leg, awkward trip and crude shunt later, we both went crashing down. But even here Mark had managed to reverse the hold upon the stick mid-fall and now pinned my arm painfully behind my back as I growled upon the frost hardened earth again.

"That was too aggressive. We're not training to be aggressive, Te is an art of non-confrontation. Try again." He was right. For some reason I was tense in both body and mind and this was reflecting into my technique. Rather than try to avoid the initial strike I'd rushed in recklessly, had there been more than one opponent I was also wide open for a counter attack.

The training session continued like this for another half hour or so with little improvement on my behalf. When the drizzle and fog rolled down the hills with a bitter bite we called it a day and went inside.

When Mark married on Okinawa it was a relative who first introduced him to Te. Uncle Saburo. For several years he'd been studying Goju-ryu, a karate style that literally means 'hard/soft' but was rapidly becoming more hard than soft by the majority of those now practising it. Uncle Saburo was known to have studied with some of the older *bujin* masters of a past generation and gradually Mark convinced him to open up more about his training whenever the chance arose. Obligingly, though reluctantly at first, Uncle Saburo passed on titbits of wisdom including a hotchpotch of breathing techniques, stretches, strikes and throws. None of which was sporty or for show but all of which was simple, subtle and direct. This was how Te was before the advent of karate 'styles', before economically hard pressed Okinawans realised their martial skills could become a viable source of income by opening commercial dojos and watering down their teachings for the masses.

In the old days the way of teaching and learning was often private, one to one, and away from prying eyes either in homes, backyards or the peaceful graveyards above the townships in the quiet of night. Contrary to the concept that it is hard to teach your own children a lot of Te was passed on from father to son, or from one generation to another as with Uncle Saburo and Mark. By the twentieth century some of the first styles of karate, kobudo and Te to emerge publicly were family traditions with lineages reaching back to the 1700's and beyond.

Mark was introduced to another family renowned on Okinawa for their martial skill; the Higa's. Teaching from a small dojo called the Bugeikan, Higa Seitoku was a *bujin* with an impressive background. From an early age he had studied a style of Tomari-te from his father, who had himself trained directly under a famous Kokan Oyadomari. Then from the age of twelve he began training under his life-long teacher Kishimoto Soko.

Kishimoto was an *Aji* feudal lord who hailed from a noble warrior clan of the Sho Dynasty Era. He taught Seitoku the Te he had learned from his own teacher Tachimura, a senior official of the Palace and a renowned *bujin* of the late 1800's. One story tells how during the turbulent period of land reforms that swept the islands Tachimura was set upon by a large gang intent on maiming him.

Witness accounts tell how Tachimura, was seen ducking and diving amidst the throng of hatchet wielding toughs avoiding their strikes as he retreated back to the boat. Occasionally he would flick up a sweeping kick which would see its victim run screaming from the affray clutching a bloody flap of skin from their head. This scalping kick was no doubt the result of a concealed blade hidden in the sole of Tachimura's shoe; for the art of concealing weapons for self-defence had long been practised on Okinawa since the 1600's. It was after this ordeal that Tachimura, then retired to the north of the island where he taught Kishimoto.

Kishimoto died during the 1945 Battle of Okinawa from a stray bullet when US forces clashed with the Imperial Japanese army and the impoverished Okinawans were caught in the crossfire. He was eighty-two and something of one of the last of the true 'old school' masters on the island.

After the war Higa Seitoku embarked upon an ambitious project to preserve as much of the wisdom from an ageing generation of martial art masters as he could. His intention was to safeguard these systems as unique cultural arts against the changing tide of 'sport based' karate then washing through the capital. Training privately and intensively for many years he eventually gained teacher and successor certificates in several styles including: Yamane ryu, Motobu Udundi, Shuri-te karate,

Tomari-te and Okinawan kobudo; all in addition to the Te he'd learnt from Kishimoto.

In fact, it was largely through his connection with the Higa family that Mark was able to meet many of the senior masters he interviewed for his first book. One such teacher was Nakama Chozo who privately taught Seitoku Higa's son, Kiyohiko as did Kanzo Nakadankari, both of whom, I would later discover, had an important influence upon the karate taught at the Bugeikan and valuably linked back to Funakoshi's early training.

Bit by bit my training was developing too. By living with Mark I came to realise that my personal work ethic was often too intense and sometimes detrimental to the final outcome.

For example if a job needed doing my inclination was always to get on and get it done. So when a new drainage ditch needed digging, because rain water from the adjacent fields was washing against the foundations of the house, I envisioned a big job and a full day of digging. I saw it as a chore but ultimately one that needed doing. However we split that job over a couple of weeks.

Another time, when we discussed thinning the woodland at the southern end of the farm, I thought a day of chopping lay ahead. Instead we did a few hours one afternoon and then came back to it once or twice a week until enough was done and next years wood pile had been stacked. Such jobs were a way of working the body physically but not to the point of exhaustion and so each day we just did a little more; bit by bit, one step at a time.

Slowly, like the tale of the hare and the tortoise, I learnt to break tasks down into smaller stages and began to see the real progress made through consistent effort. Of course, learning martial arts is just like this, you don't run before you walk, you learn a few fundamentals and then build upon them.

The manual work about the farm was physical and gave a good workout whereas compiling the books became a mental exercise with the mind active and body inactive. Our Te training became the spiritual aspect that brought a wholesome balance to the trinity of body, mind and soul. Living on the farm became an almost monastic experience but one spared of dogma and scripture. It was true zen.

11
Letting Go
"Attachment is the root of all suffering"

During my time in France Mark and I would often exchange shiatsu sessions to relieve the aches from training and release the karmic tensions being exorcised through the writing down of memories and reliving of past experiences.

My connection with Mark had always been a comfortable one but I am aware that others in the martial arts world have expressed difficulty and wariness in his presence. In many ways Mark is a mirror through which one can observe, albeit on a subconscious level, positive and negative traits within themselves. He is not the sort of teacher one often encounters these days and as such the intensity of his persona has a tendency to serve as a catalyst for great change. My observation has been that people who speak derogatory of him are usually awash with fear. Not a fear of the man himself but a fear of change.

In shiatsu terms it is not unheard of for recipients of treatment to later break-up from their partners, leave a career or embark on new adventures that friends and family might see as 'out of character'. A lot of people in the world are unhappy in their lives, un-nourished or feel trapped by circumstances surrounding the relationships they are in. Such individuals tend to hide their insecurities behind masks and barriers in order to keep the status quo and avoid rocking the boat. Over a prolonged period of time this can lead to sickness and disease which shiatsu technique will look to release. In many ways it can be said that Mark's expression of 'being' is what often lights the fuse that starts the process which brings these changes about. Shiatsu of course being just one method, martial arts another, writing another and painting too.

The truth is we learn more from the things that cause us emotional pain than we do from being comfortable, and so in order to reap the full potential of this life experience we must always strive to embrace new encounters, forgive the wrong doings of others, be grateful for what we have and move towards the things that drive us. Harbouring resentment, guilt and fear only ever leads to sickness and disease. The transformative wisdom of life arts such as Te, karate and shiatsu empowers people to overcome these afflictions and reach their full potential on a holistic level. It's the journey to enlightenment; a state of being where sickness cannot reside in the body for it finds no purchase in the mind. This is the real purpose of the life arts.

Ask different people their impression of Mark and you'll likely get different answers. But then isn't that true of all of us?

For some people though it is the way he looks, or rather 'sees'. During my time living with him I witnessed this frequently. Every couple of weeks we would make the drive to town to stock up on food and necessities. On these trips I became aware of the way people, other drivers, strangers on the side of the road, or customers in shops, would suddenly stop their conversations and become transfixed on Mark's presence. Their faces would seem to change, sometimes demonically, to an expression of what I could only describe as hatred.

It sounds ridiculous and far fetched but it was, nonetheless, observable. The first time I noticed it was in the airport. Mark was sitting eating a sandwich and a man from across the other side of the departure lounge locked onto him and literally scowled, apropos of nothing. Of course at first I half suspected he had recognised him from some previous encounter but when similar things were happening wherever we travelled I felt this couldn't always be the case. Most of the time I don't even think Mark was aware of it happening at all, which just made the attention he gained even more bizarre to witness.

Another time a senior trainee admitted to me that after a session with Mark he felt 'odd' and somewhat 'uncomfortable' with the day's events. Though he could not fault the martial content of the class he distinctly felt that when Mark looked at him, he was being fully read like an open book, as if his most closely kept secrets were on display. It made me think of the Grandmaster in Japan and the teacher of the fanatical group that followed him. But in comparison I would say that where they, for me at least, represented a certain darkness, Mark was light. I never once witnessed him act maliciously or negatively to anyone. When he probed or influenced a situation he did so to kickstart a chain of events that although might at first seem disruptive and hugely destructive would ultimately bring about a positive change of circumstance for the better. Much like how a zen monk might offer some paradoxical phrase to induce a paradigm shift in an acolyte's thinking. Thus clearing away the clouds of the mind.

Like the 'polished' mirror state idealised in karate, it was as if when people looked at Mark the darkest aspects of their own psyche were reflected back at them even if for just a fleeting moment. Nevertheless this process of change, which amounts to an emancipation of sorts, is rarely easy to endure and naturally a large part of the work must of course be borne out by the one experiencing the change themselves.

In some way my work as a shiatsu therapist, built upon the experiences of my past, meant I understood all this long before I arrived in France and so naturally I was expecting a certain level of turmoil to follow in the duration of my stay. It was, after all, just one more sacrifice amongst many that I had made to experience the type of teaching I was pursuing.

For me personally a lot of my karmic issues surfaced at night. My dreams in those early weeks were vivid and wild, tormented by fierce storms, hurricanes and whirling crashing sounds, coupled with notions of being pulled from my body and flung endlessly through skies and heavens above. But it was the failed relationships with ex-girlfriends that haunted me in a more wicked way.

Regularly I would wake peacefully with visions that past romances were still very much alive and in the height of the 'good days' only to suddenly realise, as my eyes flickered open to an empty pillow, that the flames of such companionship had long been extinguished and I was essentially alone. Morning after morning this torment occurred like a visit to purgatory leaving me feeling the washed out, empty feelings of a recently broken heart. This melancholy self-doubt then set the day ahead and this kind of tribulation lasted several weeks. Of course at the time I'd keep such thoughts private and use my training to release the anguish as best I could but while on the surface I tried to remain unaffected I'm certain this veneer did not really fool anyone.

It didn't matter. The whole purpose of our training was to 'let go'. The mind, body and spirit form a matrix of health and martial arts is just one way to achieve balance within this trinity. Physical training is required because our reality is to experience the three-dimensional world we live in through our senses. The body, essentially a vehicle for the soul, needs to be strong and healthy so early training focusses on the perfection of stances and dynamics of movement. The breath is the bridge between the physical and mental aspects of this matrix and with clear breathing comes clarity of thought. After all, the mind and body are not separate but one and troubles of the mind, if left unchecked, will impair physical health just as sickness and injury will affect mental wellbeing too. Spiritual good health is reflected in a mind free from attachment and fixed ideas. You have to let go of the past. Open the body up and the mind will follow.

✽

"Pick a weapon. And another. One more. Okay. Lets train spiritually."

It was early January the following year and wrapped up in winter coats, hats, scarves and boots we made our way to the dojo outside. Pausing by the collection of training weapons under the eaves of the veranda I settled for a four-foot staff, a wooden sword and a pair of *tonfa*.

Yesterday's rain had left the ground underfoot sodden and treacherous as Mark and I practised *bukitori*, the skill of reclaiming a weapon from an opponent. In ancient times *bukitori* enabled a warrior to stay in the battle following the unfortunate event of his own weapon being lost or broken. Today the methods remain useful in disarming would-be attackers running at you with sticks, bottles or knives.

A lot of our early *kumite* training focussed heavily upon the classical weaponry forms of Te such as the bow, sword, glaive and spear. Mostly this coincided with each chapter of Okinawan Weaponry then being polished for the final print. Although such weapons are rarely encountered on the streets today they continue to teach many skills relevant to empty hand technique. For example the bow or *'yumi'* teaches about expansion and contraction, the spear about fast piercing thrusts along linear angles, and the *naginata* about slicing and sphericity of movement. Perhaps more than any other martial art Te is like this.

As we stood now with a light rain falling upon our faces I wondered why Te, a supposed non-confrontational martial art, centred so heavily upon weaponry training and I'd questioned Mark about its spiritual justification because it had been clouding my mind for several days.

"Physically, in Te, we train to avoid all strikes and simply enter a situation passively." Mark gripped the handle of the wooden sword he'd taken from me moments earlier and adopted the subtlest of stances. To an onlooker he might not have looked like he was ready to attack, but he was.

"We do not cause confrontation. Confrontation is when one thing blocks the way of another. In life we extend this principle to the manner in which we speak and deal with others - we do not clash or suppress but rather guide and nurture. In Te we yield to oncoming force and redirect it just as we do in life. Therefore weaponry training leads to spiritual development."

Nodding, I scanned for an opening. Non-confrontation is a core principle of Te and one that was adopted successfully as the former Ryukyu Kingdom's foreign policy. Surrounded by Japan, China and Korea, Okinawan kings applied a non-confrontational approach to existing with their powerful neighbours but without being bullied by them. A bit like Switzerland does today. I imagine that this concept of 'pacifism' originated from early South Pacific peoples use of natural ocean currents, trade winds and stars to accurately plot courses between the specks of land jutting from the Pacific with just the crudest of craft and equipment. Such early navigators learnt to read the subtle clues of cloud and wave formations which signalled to them their proximity to land, even if it could not yet be seen by eye. Another term for pacifism is 'going with the flow'.

There was a pause, a battle of wills, the time-gap between inaction and action.
In a flash the heavy *bokken* 'whomped' down towards my head. Instinctively I darted forward on a diagonal entry twisting to avoid the cut and simultaneously slipping my hand along the inside of Mark's wrist to close about the weapon's hilt. Was it now his sword or mine?
Turning on the spot my body merged with the flow of his attack and I tried to lock his elbow against my flank. Sensing this Mark drove it sharply towards my ribs. My body sculpted to avoid the strike and I jabbed at his face. Like a dance, albeit an un-choreographed one, Mark's footwork enabled him to turn the blade back towards me destroying my counter-attack no sooner than it'd begun. Seeing a new opening, a weakly positioned arm, I seized upon the hilt with both hands and tried

to wrench the sword from him. I gritted my teeth and tugged hard but rather than wrestle, he let go of the weapon altogether. Confusion. The sword was now firmly in both my hands, but like a prank of someone opening a door just as you are about to forcefully push it from the other side my zealous actions had left me totally vulnerable.

Clutching the weapon with two hands I was unable to defend as Mark thrust his thumbs into my throat and ribs. My posture crumbled and jaw clenched. Releasing one hand I tried to punch again but he deftly avoided this and re-gripped the hilt of the weapon trapping my remaining hand to it. When I pulled the weapon close, in an attempt to break his hold, the blade was turned upon me. Trapped, I couldn't let go even if I wanted to.

"Attachment is the root of all suffering."

Mark grinned as his blue eyes drew my attention to his grip upon the *bokken*. The match was won. Had it been a real sword the cutting edge would have swept back under my own arm severing the tendons that enabled me to hold it. Instead, a large suffocating hand clutched about my face, turning me aside as he reclaimed full control of the weapon and brought it back in a cleaving two-handed cut that stopped half an inch above me.

The whole thing probably took less than a few seconds. Had this been on a battlefield I'd be dead. Where I went wrong was thinking I needed to hold the weapon to be in control of it. But the sword was only the illusion of power, an inanimate object that is only really powerful when wielded expertly. In defence it's the attacker that needs to be controlled, not the weapon.

Primitively, despite my training, I had 'lost myself' in the 'heat of battle' and had resorted to using muscular strength to try and succeed. I believe riot police are prone to the same when facing an aggressive crowd. Armed with shield and baton they 'know', intellectually, that jabbing the stick in linear fashion is the most effective use of the truncheon. But very often, when it all 'kicks off', you see them slip back into using caveman clubbing strikes. Like a person with a short-temper suddenly they are 'beside them self' possessed by a snorting animal ready to rampage. Lose the plot. Go ape. Flip. Through training in Te we strive to rise above base behaviours like these, which in itself is the essence of spiritual training.

Rather than try to wrestle the weapon from Mark's grip I should have simply let go and expanded with empty hands. Karate means 'empty hand' but really it is the mind that must be emptied. It's all so easy in theory. So logical. The real challenge is putting things into practice.

Training sessions like these offer the opportunity to develop yourself spiritually because you learn from your mistakes, the little deaths and rebirths of *kumite* matches.

In the years before living with Mark I'd often taken to wild camping in the foothills of either Mt. Snowdonia in Wales or along the 'Pilgrims Path' of the Pyrenees. The purpose of these excursions, which could last weeks or months, were to train alone in nature and focus introspectively upon the lessons I'd learnt from my experiences in Japan. Lessons from The Group, The Grandmaster and the Old Man, each of whose words echoed in my mind long after I had met them. Despite the real progress made unlocking the methods of Funakoshi's karate through kata during my early experimentations, it was ultimately my footwork that prevented me making the real advances needed to elevate my techniques to the next level.

In Te, which literally means 'hands', it is the hands that are the medium by which you engage with an opponent's incoming attack, but it is the footwork that truly enables you to enter, unbalance and neutralise the attack. When a hopeful student approached a famous Te master for instruction he was told 'I can't teach you Te because you learn with your feet.'

Likewise despite recognising the T-stance of Funakoshi's approach the photographs and illustrations of his books ultimately revealed it to be a rooted posture, when in fact the aim is to rise on to the balls of the feet with heels lifted. In Te the same stance is called "*tachugwa*" or 'rising to the summit' pose.

In addition to training in Te on Okinawa, Mark had also studied traditional dance under the private tuition of a theatre teacher. Classical dance footwork is slow and meditative. It is reflective of old 'Court Culture' and in his autobiography Funakoshi had made frequent reference to his insistence of adopting this 'old fashioned' walking style throughout his entire life. I feel it was another breadcrumb clue left behind for those 'searching for the old' because in all other aspects Funakoshi felt compelled to hide Ryukyuan culture. if you were to take the time to look into the origins of this 'out dated' walking style you wouldn't stumble into Shuri erudite culture, you'd literally stride elegantly right into the heart of it.

In Te, for combat, the footwork lightens up and comes alive. One of the biggest hurdles for karate-ka approaching Te is its very liberated footwork. It's also one of the factors that really strengthens the argument that Te was a distinct martial art. With heels lifted, and knees too, the basic movement forms comprise of skips and shuffles similar at first to *kendo* fencing. Then there are side shuffles, turns and jumps as well. The practicality behind this method is two fold. Firstly it makes it difficult for an opponent to read your own movement with regards to advancing. Secondly it enables you to keep ever mobile and fluid to respond to any type of attack. Anchoring the feet to the ground in Te is called 'dead stance' for the simple reason you will become like a sitting duck.

This was highlighted to Mark in Okinawa when his teacher took a bokken sword and swung it down towards his head. Instinctively, at the time, having been trained in Goju-ryu karate, Mark anchored his feet, adopted a strong stance and thrust his forearm above his head to block. Fortunately the sword strike was pulled off to save any bruising but had it been a real sword it would have cleaved him in two. Non-confrontation means not getting in the way of superior force and Te's footwork is an agile expression of this notion. The trick is to avoid and enter into an attack simultaneously as one action as opposed to the usual 'block' then 'attack' functioning of karate proper.

In a rare photograph of Funakoshi defending from an attack at a demonstration it is clear to see him light on his feet with both heels lifted as one hand 'checks' the incoming attack and the other reaches forward to strike the attacker. Avoid and enter. One movement. This is the foundation of Te.

12
Goodbye
'Needle and thread sensei'

By Spring the following year my time with Mark was naturally coming to an end. In the dojo the buds had opened and lush green grass now reclaimed the muddy smears and scrapes of our winter training. The book projects were completed, as were most of the larger jobs about the farm. Our training routine continued much the same with morning jogs, stretching on the veranda and going at each other with sticks and swords throughout the late afternoons. My technique had come to a new level and although I felt very much alive there was a yearning inside for something more.

One day, Moya, who lived with Mark and brought a grounded sense of stability to the farm and our life there, was coming out of the supermarket pushing a trolley of groceries. From the backseat of the car I had noticed a group of drunks loitering and harassing other women leaving the store, so I told Mark, who was sitting in the front, to watch out for her.

His eyes scanned the five men across the parking lot and with a nod he went to meet her just as one of them was attempting to take control of her trolley. I had no real concern for my sensei, the group was intimidating but heavily intoxicated. Nonetheless I watched from the side of the car. I didn't want to inflame things by also approaching but remained ever ready to rush in if needed. Besides, I was intrigued to see how he would handle this.

Striding confidently towards the man holding onto the trolley Mark clapped his hands as if scarring away a stray dog and took him completely by surprise. The drunkard's four friends stirred tentatively and lurched from their place by the railings.

Taking the trolley I watched as Mark subtly positioned himself between the group, with Moya behind him, and thrust it forwards with a motion to encourage the man away. Separated from his pack he backed towards a stack of other trolleys and tripped over. Some of the group tried to move in on Mark, baffled but perhaps rilled as to what was going on. With a stern finger he pointed accusingly at them with a scolding glare that scattered them away as if invisible thunder bolts were about to shoot forth from his hand. The situation was over. No one was hurt and no one had the stomach to continue. As they went to help their friend from the ground a security guard came over and told them all to leave.

It wasn't a fight. But it was a confrontation that had the potential to escalate. Mark's response highlighted a lesson I'd learnt long before whilst managing an inner city bar. That lesson was that being out numbered needn't equate to being at a disadvantage. When there is a group involved there is a whole different dynamic that can be played, directed and influenced. Few want to be the first to rush in on a competent and confident fighter so there are usually waves of advances and retreats both verbal and physical. In the end psychological tactics will always play a greater part. They need to have an appetite for it, and groups are rarely looking to start trouble on a capable fighter; why risk it when there are always softer targets to victimise.

Getting back into the car I noticed Mark's eyes were sharp and clear. But not in the usual sense of the phrase though. There was a different intensity.

I'd witnessed this twice before and had made reference to it in my journal. The best way for me to describe it is as though he had dark eye-liner makeup on. The eyelids themselves seemed keen and cutting serving to make the whites of his eyes appear wide and glaring. I might also add it lent a certain 'non-human' quality to his aura. Classical Indian artwork also depicts noble warriors and demigod's with similar eyes. I used to think it implied the use of makeup but now I believe it is the artists rendition of witnessing this same phenomena. Mark was not wearing eye-liner and, like the times before, the appearance subsided within a few minutes.

It is, I have come to realise, a technique of sorts.

The iconic front cover images of Gichin Funakoshi's books *Karate-Dō Kyohan* and *Nyumon* portray two of the Guardian King statues of Buddhism. Zocho-ten is the Guardian of the South and his expression is a fierce glare with wide eyes, flared nostrils and curled lips; the embodiment of power released. Komoku-ten, the Guardian of the West, carries the expression of power held in reserve. His brow is creased with eyes narrowed and nostrils slightly pinched with indignation. The remaining two statues carry expressions of a similar vein as they stand upon demonic dog-like beasts which glance upwards in surrendered fear of their conquerors.

The four glares aren't taught in modern karate but they are taught in Te and I'm certain Funakoshi well understood the significance of them too. To understand the power of such expressions is to understand the human response to fear and stress. Adrenaline.

Body language accounts for nearly ninety percent of the way we communicate with one another and all mammals engage in staring as a demonstration of antagonistic behaviour when defending mating or territory rights. In potential fight situations the stare-down is a strategy adopted to attain victory without resorting to physical fighting, which in itself carries potential risks to survival from injury. The stare down then is a psychological battle that ultimately seeks to cause the opponent to doubt their own ability and crumble from within. Shouting, or the karate *kiai*, is an extension of this.

Therefore fighting is not only ethically the last resort but instinctively the least favoured too. When the brain perceives a threat it stimulates the secretion of hormones that instantly trigger a number of changes in the body. Some of these changes include rapid breathing to oxygenate the blood, an elevated heart rate to prepare the body for strenuous activity and the release of other hormones to lower the pain threshold. Additionally the function of the digestive tract is shut down to further conserve energy whilst circulation is also withdrawn from the outer extremities where it becomes concentrated in the torso and limbs.

Such responses, induced under threat, are instinctively given an intensity appropriate to the individual's requirements and can empower them to run from, or fight, the source of that threat. It is commonly referred to as the 'fight or flight' response but in actuality this term is both incorrect and back to front. There are really three phases that escalate from first to last depending on the intensity of the situation; freeze, flight or fight.

Fighting is instinctively the least preferred response to aggression because self-preservation is the primary motivator. Most predators in the animal kingdom target their intended prey by tracking movement, therefore the ability to remain absolutely still, freeze, is an instinctive trait that evolved millions of years ago. During this phase the sense gathering organs help intuit the brain to assess the risks and make a decision to either run or fight. This calculation is fast and more informed than rational thinking. Sometimes the body shuts down through an overload of fear giving the appearance of death, just like when someone faints.

Many people who have survived an attack or extreme threat are able to recount the minutest of details, and make the retelling of an incident that took less than ten seconds last many minutes. This is because a particular part of the brain, the amygdala, is basing its assessment not only on the information gathered from all the senses but also from previous experiences and memories including ancestral ones held in the DNA, karma. Gaining conscious control of the amygdala leads to a state of enhanced situational awareness known in martial arts as *zanshin*.

If 'freezing' and blending with the environment are not conducive to survival then taking flight, that is 'running away', becomes the next preferred option. The secretion of adrenaline enables the muscles of the legs to sprint-start and maintain a considerable pace for an extended period of time. Added with the state of increased awareness described from the 'freeze' phase, people are able to traverse rough and uneven ground with apparent greater dexterity than normal so as to avoid a trip or fall that could have detrimental results.

Finally, if freezing or fleeing are not likely to lead to the best chance of survival then the individual under threat will lash out to defend themselves. Fight.

Continued training in martial arts develops a stillness of mind in the face of adversity so that one can remain calm and 'level-headed' in heated situations. Real training then is not to suppress natural or instinctive responses of the human experience but to acknowledge and accept them as the primitive reactions they are, and then harness them into a decisive response. When coupled with trained responses, utilising good body-dynamics and a clear mind, the result is an individual able to tackle multiple opponents both armed and unarmed. A reasonable definition of the term warrior, or *bushi*.

Serious *bujin* should contemplate what this means and teachers should consider the wider consequences of their teachings. Failure to recognise, familiarise and reconcile with the effects of the freeze, flight or fight response will significantly reduce an individuals ability to capture and harness this potential energy. Worst still it can cause confusion in the mind and sap morale and confidence to the point it will negatively destroy the individual from within.

For example during a violent situation it is not uncommon to experience body shaking, trembling hands, cold-sweats, a racing heart and a quivering voice. Socially these traits are commonly associated with fear and weakness but in fact they are just side-effects of the hormonal changes taking place in response to the threat. Lingering in this jittery state further builds anxiety and the clouded mind will begin to throw up moral dilemma's 'is it right or wrong?', 'what if I fail?', 'Can I really win?'.

At such times you must remember to come into the *hara*, exhale and let go.

When the focus of martial arts shifts away from the competition arena and is instead realigned with the goals of health development and self-preservation then understanding human behaviour becomes essential for progression. More than this, it enables the advanced *bujin* to gain a keen insight into reading the subtle dynamics or 'tells' in both people and situations.

The Four Glares provide a method upon which to maintain self control whilst facing adversity, whilst simultaneously inspiring fear and doubt in an opponent.

How do they work? Each expression displayed by the Heavenly Kings referenced in Funakoshi's books and tales of his teacher Matusmura, is a glare that can be applied to different circumstances. Zocho-ten is the release of power likened to a fierce battle cry in the heat of conflict. It's purpose is to invoke fear and routing. Komoku-ten's expression, as mentioned earlier, is the look of power held in reserve. His face is serious but calm as if assessing the situation and quietly 'judging'. He does not give much away leaving the opponent questioning and doubting.

The other statues display the emotions of disgusted indignation and resentment. Indignation is expressed against those deemed to be of a perceived lower social level than our own. They project feelings of reduced self-worth and shame. The nostrils are pinched, lips pursed and eyes lifted to the corners with the brow shaped like the letter V.

Whereas indignation is expressed to those lower than ourselves, resentment is the emotion reserved for those of a higher perceived social standing. Eyes narrowed, lips pursed and lifted at one corner, the final statue expresses contempt and resentment.

There are of course other facial expressions of emotion that were known within the Ryukyu Kingdom era which related more to influencing positive business relations with others. The power of the smiles to make others feel at ease should not be underestimated either. Such expressions or 'mimes' have been preserved in a number of the *kumiodori* performances of traditional Okinawan theatre and would certainly have been known by a performer such as Funakoshi's father.

After the event in the carpark I came to understand that Mark was also well versed in these expressions too, which probably accounted for the strange looks he would get from strangers sometimes.

*

The final chapters of *Okinawan Weaponry* had dealt largely with the clandestine weapons of Te. Pocket knives, parasols, paper fans and even hairpins were all discreet self-defence weapons carried by the 'gentlemen of Shuri' during the days of the Ryukyu Kingdom. More obscure items included the simple hand-towel, chopsticks and smoking pipes.

Our Te training reflected this as best we could utilising small hand held items to apply pressure to *tsubo* points whilst escaping from various close range grabs and tackles. With such training a new sense of self-confidence blossomed and I found myself walking about in a state of blissful awareness. A state of existence in which I had no concerns of being attacked or caught unawares.

Over the years I've met so many instructors of karate who make a point of not sitting with their backs to doorways, giving corners a wide berth or generally going about their days in a state of near paranoia from potential attacks. As if the whole world is a potential enemy. I've come to realise that the harbouring of such thought patterns is more likely to transmute them into their physical reality than not. Just as conditioning the hands and feet to be effective weapons will do the same. Each and every one of us is creating our own karma.

The heightened state of awareness I was now experiencing felt natural. Both invigorating and calm. It was like a sense of 'knowing' that, should an attack occur, what will be will be. After all, karate, Te or any martial art, can never guarantee the outcome of an engagement anyway. At best we can hope it improves our odds of survival, but for low level styles the opposite is also true.

True martial arts training is about putting health first and then the combative aspects really become a by-product of this. The rationale is simple. Unless you are in a profession where you are required to face violence on a daily basis then 'fighting' shouldn't be the primary motivation for your training. If you train week in and week out solely for that possible 'once in a lifetime encounter' then you are suffering from paranoia. More than this, the stress of carrying around all that unspent adrenaline will tax your immune system and lead to reduced health. Traditional martial arts training provides a means to release these toxins, which we accumulate enough of through modern living.

Back on the farm, despite the calmness of Spring and the sun drenched days on the veranda, a certain restlessness was stirring. Mark was keen to travel to another property in the south and, in the absence of larger jobs to be completed during the days, I had taken to hiking over the hills and exploring further afield. I was welcomed to stay and look after the place until he returned in the Autumn but a burning desire was forming in my heart and I knew the time was coming for me to move on too. There was something I had to experience for myself. Someone I had to meet.

About three years before coming out to Mark I had suffered an illness that had me bed bound for several weeks. During this time a great many changes were taking place in my body on a cellular level as I suffered from constant fevers and hallucinations. Towards the end of this period, for roughly ten days, I found myself waking from a repetitive dream at exactly

03:15 each morning. In this dream I played a passive role witnessing a man dressed in white *hakama* and kimono defending against multiple attackers wielding spears, swords and staffs. His movements were graceful and fluid, fearless and liberated as he effortlessly tossed each assailant away in a swirl of movement and remained untouched. When I woke from these dreams I wanted to record the movements in my journal but found the usual 'stickman' figures I usually used for this purpose too static and stiff to truly convey what I saw.

Determined to record the techniques in some form I dragged myself from bed and went out into the garden to rehearse them over and over until the clarity of the vision faded. If at any point I felt that 'I' was influencing the next movement I'd stop and return to bed. After a few days a kata of sorts was forming, and when the form eventually came to an end my sickness had fully subsided. In my mind I linked the significance of these dreams to the one I'd had years before after training with the Old Man, the dream in which I climbed a mountain path and awoke with that lingering vibration.

In the front of Mark's fourth book, *Zen Odyssey*, I had succeeded in convincing him to include a piece of brushwork art from his *sempai* in Okinawa, Higa Kiyohiko. My reasons were somewhat selfish.

Sometimes in life, perhaps only a few times, you experience a moment where intuitively something 'clicks' and everything seems right. An omen. Perhaps you meet a person, see something profound in the mundane, or have the sensation that this was just, 'meant to be'; a waypoint on a long journey that makes you smile and think, 'no matter how tough things might be, or have been, or how lost and uncertain you feel, you are exactly where you are meant to be. The right time. The right place. A private message that guides you towards your destiny. Such feelings are not really rational or logical but speak directly to your heart.

When I first found that painting, rolled up as it was amidst a collection of artwork and certificates, I had that distinct feeling. I took it to be a sign.

So powerful were the emotions stirring in my heart that I suggested the piece should be included in the book. The piece didn't really hold any great significance to the book itself, and the copy that appears in no way does the original justice, but that didn't really matter I wanted it included because I wanted a copy for future reference.

The reason was that although I'd never seen the painting before I had seen the place it portrayed. I'd been there. In a dream. "That's the place." I said to myself as I plucked it from the collection of documents from Mark's travels.

A jungle forest covered mountain, rich with vegetation and an aura of power, approached by a single meandering path; an arduous journey with a sense of purpose and destiny. The painting wasn't just 'like' that place in my dream, from all those years ago, it 'was' that place.

Of course the painting was really just a figment of the artists' mind. Not a life composition taken in the field or reproduced from some earlier sketches but created free-form, without constraint. Pure creation. Divinely inspired.

The accompanying kanji inscription read: '*Seisei Jōjō*', 'quietly, gracefully, purely'.

The thoughts that formed in my mind threaded that early dream and its waking reality with the repetitive dreams of the man dressed in a white kimono. That man now had a name. Higa Kiyohiko. And I was ready to embark upon the next stage of my martial arts journey.

Unlike most sensei Mark does not use the terms 'student' or 'disciple'. Instead he says 'trainee' and likens the role of a sensei to the eye of a needle; the trainee is the thread. It was this sense of 'non attachment', 'non-ownership' that had become the second marker by which I gauged a teacher worth training with over the years.

One evening, standing on the veranda gazing out to the Pyrenees, painted as they were in a red haze from the setting sun, I recalled with melancholy that whenever I found a good sensei, circumstance or Fate it seemed, would dictate that they would not be around for long. Most of the time I preferred things this way, 'drink deeply' and then retreat away to contemplate and 'own' the lesson's I'd been taught slowly and patiently at my own pace. Sometimes though it had made for a lonely journey and felt like wandering in the dark.

Mark however thought it was a healthy way to be.

"Stay with a teacher too long and you will pick up their bad habits." And so it was, with a knowing nod and unspoken sadness, we headed to the car and drove to the airport. This chapter in my training had come to end.

13
Okinawa
'Island of martial arts'

Through the small round window I could see the southern islands of Yonaguni, Yaeyama and Ishigaki far below shaded by a train of cotton-candy clouds. The Ryukyu Islands span 750 miles between Japan and Taiwan and are divided into the three groups of Southern, Central and Northern by two expanses of sea known as the Kerama Gap and Tokara Straits. In a short while I'd be flying over the later and landing in Naha.

Before the last glacial period the islands were linked to the Asian continent by land bridges but as sea levels rose about 12,000 years ago the inhabitants became isolated and unique cultures emerged. Despite the humid sub-tropical climate of the region some of the oldest human remains ever discovered in Asia have been found in the Ryukyu's, lending further weight to the theory that humanity, technology and mathematics spread from the Pacific peoples to the estuaries of major rivers and coastal regions around the world.

No sooner had we taken off it seemed we were descending again. Half an hour later, with a bag over my shoulder, I set out to embark upon my Okinawan adventure.

As far as cities go Naha has a sort of surreal 'theme park' quality to it that reminded me of a childhood visit to Disney World. Streets were clean and despite the hustle and bustle of traffic the feeling in the air was fresh and lively. The sidewalks seemed crowded with pretty girls walking by in mini-skirts and tube-socks while plinky cartoon-like tunes played from brightly coloured shopfronts and the monorail hummed overhead weaving through the city. Unlike my first arrival in Tokyo, all those years ago, Naha at once felt like home and I had an uncanny sense of direction which required no maps to find my way around. Deep down inside I felt more at home there than anywhere else I've ever been in the world.

From the airport I made my way to 'Koksai Dori', 'International Street'. Nearby was the Eager Beaver bar, which an acquaintance in England suggested I visit to meet with the owner and gain a contact on the ground. The bar was closed so I made my way through town towards Naminoue Beach where I intended to check into a hostel for my first few nights.

BASE Okinawa was a soft flamingo pink building tucked into the backstreets around Naha's 'red-light' district of Tsuji. It was run that season by a friendly young crowd of Japanese, most of whom had travelled to Okinawa from the mainland to work in its tourist industry or to cut sugar cane in the farms to the south. I settled for a dormitory room with an on-suite bathroom shared between four. It was cramped but it was clean and it didn't break the bank.

Keen to get training as quickly as I could I set out to find the Bugeikan. I had jotted down the address in a leather bound notebook but when I found the place there was nothing there but a rusting 1950's American car on an overgrown building plot nestled at the crossroad of a busy intersection. Mark had long been out of contact with the Higa's and so this journey was totally off my own back and somewhat blind. The address had come from an old directory I'd found and with nothing to suggest a dojo nearby I wandered aimlessly searching for clues and waiting for inspiration.

Down a side street not far away another one of those signs came to me. I began to experience a tangible vibration that resonated in my chest and spread to my fingers and toes. It wasn't uncomfortable and I accepted it as instinct telling me I must be close, but where? Ultimately I couldn't find a dojo of any sorts and so somewhat disheartened I eventually gave up and rode the monorail back through town hoping that the Eager Beaver might now be open for lunch. It wasn't. Instead I came upon the famous martial arts shop Shureido and had a look at the various kobudo weapons and books for sale.

After a conversation with the owner of the store he obligingly called an old number for the Higa's on my behalf. After the Second World War Higa Seitoku had been a driving force in the popularisation of martial arts on the island and Shureido was 'the' shop for clothing and equipment. However after a brief conversation he set the phone back upon the receiver and sadly shook his head.

"Higa sensei no longer teaches martial arts and the Bugeikan is closed. I'm very sorry, but you've come all this way for nothing." So close and yet so far, I nodded and left.

'No' was not going to be an answer I could afford to accept. Not after everything I had been through in my quest to learn more about Okinawan martial arts and the origins of karate and Te. My one consuming desire had been to meet Mr Higa for so long that that was exactly what I intended to do, even if it meant door-stopping him. All I had to do was find out where he lived.

After a light lunch in a noodle bar I headed back to the area where I had that tingling sensation, but by late afternoon I had walked in circles throughout the neighbourhood without success. Occasionally I'd ask passersby if they knew a dojo around but none did. I looked for karate-ka wearing *gi's* making their way to a lesson but there were none. As evening set in I was about to head back to the hostel when, as a last ditch attempt, I asked a man pulling into his driveway. He nodded enthusiastically "Get in my car and I will take you there." This seemed too good to be true, and despite his best intentions it turned into a wild goose chase of sorts.

Parking by the spot where the old car was rotting on the empty site he got out and approached the building next to it. There, at the top of a flight of concrete steps, he led me to a dojo with hanging punch bags and a few young trainees sparring in gloves and headgear. An old man came to the door and chatted for a while. I knew at once this wasn't the right place but I had to wait and see the outcome. At the mention of 'Higa' the old man shook his head and flashed a surreptitious glance in my direction. Leaning close he told our middle-man something that made the situation somewhat awkward. At length my new found guide turned with a dire expression,

"Oh dear" he stumbled along, "it seems that... Mr Higa has... died. There is no-more Bugeikan dojo. I'm very sorry."

I smiled and nodded. Probably not the response they were expecting. I knew the karate teacher must have been thinking of Higa Seitoku. After all, Shureido had spoken to someone earlier. So I pressed the good samaritan to enquire about the son, Higa Kiyohiko, and although body language alone told me this old man knew of him, he shook his head and said he did not. Instead he gave my guide new instructions and minutes later we were off again driving through Naha.

When the car came to a halt I blinked and immediately recognised the white rendered outer walls and gate from an old promotional flyer for kobudo. This wasn't the Bugeikan but the Bunbukan, a model dojo for the practise of Okinawan kobudo. My guide jumped out and excitedly pressed the intercom buzzer despite my politest protests that this definitely wasn't the place I was looking for. Nevertheless the gate was opened by an immaculately dressed gentleman wearing a traditional kimono and *hakama*, sporting a perfectly groomed white beard. This was Nakamoto sensei, a well known and respected teacher of kobudo who had written a book on the subject and had been invited to teach the art in China; something he considered a monumental honour.

My guide gone, I walked with Nakamoto on a private, 'out of hours' tour of the dojo and his personal 'kobudo museum' above it. His English was of a high level with calm mannerisms coupled with a sense of a*mour propre* that lent an air of superiority to his aura. The museum itself amounted to a large room with a central table and various posters, newspaper clippings, pictures, trophies and assorted weapons lining the walls. As we moved along these displays he called out their names. "*Tonfa, nunchaku, kama…*"

Occasionally an accompanying photo next to the item suggested its possible source of origin. Side-handled batons might have come from the handles of grindstones for milling. The nunchaku flail was possibly part of a horse bridle and bit.

Perhaps, after my time with Mark compiling '*Okinawan Weaponry*', none of the weapons on display seemed to fit their suggested origin which had all been well researched for Mark's book during the fifteen years he stayed on the islands. And equally tested for practicality in our training sessions in France. The idea that Okinawan kobudo items like these had evolved from agricultural tools is a persistent theory from a time when early writers on karate romantically depicted Okinawan farmers as the formulators of karate. The truth of course was that farmers neither had the time nor inclination to dabble in martial arts which was ultimately the luxurious pursuit of sons from wealthy merchant and warrior families in the capital.

In comparison to kobudo, Te has no weaponry kata, at least not in the conventional sense, so the training is always *kumite* driven. Kobudo, which is often taught alongside karate, is largely kata based and any *kumite* is mostly pre-arranged in that both the attacker and defender know what to expect. This lends kobudo a very polished appearance not too dissimilar to a village folk dance except in kobudo an exponent will also learn how to strike effectively with the weapon and not just do movements 'for show'. Additionally, although such items as *tonfa*, *nunchaku* and *kama* are used within Te training, their application is usually different; the *tonfa* is held by the longer shaft rather than the short right-angled handle, and the *nunchaku* is swirled differently too. Of course, aside from these more 'Chinese influenced' weapons Te predominantly utilised bladed instruments such as the sword, spear, glaive and bow.

Further along the kobudo exhibition a paper parasol rested upon a cabinet complete with a short Japanese *tanto* dagger crudely bound to its handle with black duct-tape. A 'clandestine' weapon from former times; albeit an improvised replica from the late seventies or eighties.

Annoyingly for me, Nakamoto sensei insisted that all of the items in his museum were genuine artefacts of historical relevance, even the mass produced plastic hair-comb that looked strikingly more like a discarded Afro-comb from a US marine in the 70's than it did an ornate Okinawan hair accessory from the 1770's.

I enquired about the absence of swords, spears and glaives. It wasn't that these bladed weapons weren't presented on display that bugged me, after all perhaps they were hard to come by, but that they weren't even represented with pictures and descriptions seemed bizarre. This was after all one of Okinawa's leading kobudo museums. However when I asked about such bladed weapons Nakamoto would simply shrug and give a curious smile. When I pressed the question again half an hour later he flatly denied that the bladed weapons I were describing ever existed on Okinawa. They certainly weren't taught in any kobudo dojo's today.

This didn't make sense. Assuming I'd misunderstood him I pointed to a hanging scroll painting behind him depicting a Shō Dynasty Ryukyuan ship teaming with archers leaning over the parapets and spear wielding troops lining the decks. But again he shook his head and declared

"None of those weapons have ever been found. This is just a painting from someone's imagination". Fascinating.

My line of questioning about bladed weapons was clearly bringing a certain amount of tension to what was otherwise a cordial, impromptu meeting. I sensed we were clashing because ultimately Nakamoto sensei publicly subscribes and actively promotes the 'official story' that Okinawa has always been a peaceful, unarmed pacifist nation, which was subdued effortlessly by the Satsuma Clan of Japan in 1609. It's a tale long told and preserved in books, videos and dojo's around the world but, as new research has been revealing for several years now, it's not entirely accurate.

The truth is that Okinawa has a long history of warfare and strife and it's economy during the Ryukyu Kingdom era was practically built upon the export of sulphur for gunpowder as well as swords, spears and other weapons for far off wars.

There are records of early Portuguese merchants reporting on the high value of Ryukyuan swords, of wars waged in the northern Ryukyu's expelling Satsuma samurai by force and punitive raids on pirate strongholds in the southern islands during China's crackdown on the *Wako* roaming the East China Sea.

Furthermore, early Okinawan kings had a near fascination with firearms long before such items ever arrived on Japanese shores. The Japanese term '*hinawaju*' or '*tanegashima*', used to describe an early matchlock musket is named after the port from which the item first arrived in 1543. Bound for a Ryukyuan trading station on the northern island of Tanegashima a Portuguese ship carrying the rifles was washed ashore in bad weather and the resident Japanese lord 'acquired' a few samples which were later reproduced on the mainland.

Much earlier, in 1466, a Ryukyuan diplomatic mission demonstrated the shock and awe of gunpowder to an un-nerved Ashikaga Shogunate in Kyoto. This event is thought to be the first display of gunpowder being used on the mainland since the Mongol invasion nearly two hundred years earlier. Despite becoming a pacifist nation in the modern era, and admirably so, Okinawa was no stranger to war.

One of the motivating reasons for the Satsuma Invasion of 1609 was to suppress Okinawa's rapid expansion into territories south of Japan, and then tax their lucrative trade with China. A little known fact is that the Satsuma Rebellion of 1877, loosely portrayed in the blockbuster movie '*The Last Samurai*', in which hardline 'traditional' warriors clash with a modern conscript

Imperial Army, was mostly funded by Satsuma's taxation of Ryukyuan trade. This is also one of the most likely sources of agricultural tools being used as weapons in civil defence too. During the rebellion Satsuma samurai actively trained peasant communities to conduct guerrilla warfare using everyday items from around the farm.

Nakamoto sensei wasn't really being obtuse when he repeatedly deflected my questions about bladed weapons. As far as he was concerned they were nothing to do with the kobudo he taught. His kobudo is rooted in the 17th century when a migrating aristocratic class relocated from Shuri and introduced 'Chinese flavoured' weaponry to the local populations of outlying towns and villages. Thus much of Okinawan kobudo today is intricately linked and shares many similarities to the folk dances that take place throughout the islands. If clarification were needed then I should have been asking about 'Ryukyuan kobujutsu' and not Okinawan kobudo; the differences to an outsider are subtle but significant.

Another item in the exhibition included a brass shakuhachi 'flute' which concealed a nasty looking blade not too dissimilar to an envelope-opener. Its solid form made it a hefty cosh, or paper weight, but it couldn't be played as a flute.

The flute had never made an appearance in Mark's *Okinawan Weaponry* presumably because he never found one in a dojo, but it was a valid item from the right timeframe. However, in a 'Te' sense, a regular flute would serve better as a discreet weapon than this brass one. For a start it could be played innocently under inspection, secondly it could be used as a short stick for jabbing pressure-points and thirdly a poisoned needle could be projected from one end with a quick 'puff' on the other.

Eventually I thanked Mr Nakamoto for his time and said goodbye. Despite telling me he was a very close friend of Mr Higa it was clear he had no intention of contacting him on my behalf and I was no closer to getting an introduction to meet him.

*

The following day I stumbled by chance upon a small museum dedicated to the Shō Dynasty Family. Located above a large department store in central Naha. The opening display read:

'The Ryukyu Kingdom was an independent principality encompassing the islands of Okinawa that endured for 450 years from 1429-1879.

The Kingdom developed flourishing trade and diplomatic relations with China, Japan, Korea and countries of South East Asia, founding a unique culture.

Shō Hashi founded the first Shō Dynasty by uniting the three kingdoms of Ryukyu, Hokuzan, Chuzan and Nanzan. He banned the stockpiling of weapons by the great clans and established Kume-mura as a settlement for the Binjin, 36-Families from Fuzhou in China.'

The exhibition continued with depictions of old maps, costume and accessories. Of particular note were the displays of three swords, with blades dating to the 14th century. *Chiyoganemaru*, *Jikane-maru* and *Chatanakiri*. Bladed weapons most certainly did exist within the Ryukyu's but a curious sense of amnesia seemed to prevent Okinawan's themselves from realising it. Perhaps Japan's extreme naturalisation policy of the past had somehow made it that, even in front of the evidence, modern day Okinawan's were unable to accept the advanced level of their former nation. As curious as it sounds I witnessed this on several occasions.

Another display board in the museum continued:

'The Second Shō Dynasty brought further improvements outside of Shuri-jo and obliged the outlying Aji to reside in the capital so as to weaken the political power of the periphery and strengthen the centre.

Closer to the modern era the keizuza was established to clarify the division between the samurai nobility and peasant classes. The samurai were obliged to settle the urban areas of Shuri, Naha and Tomari and the commoners were to occupy rural lands.'

This move is what ultimately led to the formation of the three township styles of karate known as Shuri-te, Naha-te and Tomari-te. The suffix of 'te' referring to the Chinese/Te hybrid that later became karate proper. Rather than the 'Te' of families hailing from those regions.

However, when one considers that Shuri, Naha and Tomari are all within walking distance of each other, and that 'martial art experts' of the day actively encouraged trainees to visit other teachers, then it becomes apparent that the stylistic differences between Shuri-te and Naha-te would have been minimal to the casual observer.

The truth behind such terms as Shuri-te, Nahate and Tomari-te is more a reflection of the social prejudices that existed in the capital of the former Ryukyuan Kingdom. And to some extent still do. It's also the reason why Shō En's restrictions on the *Aji* have perhaps played a greater influence upon karate's development than the weapon bans of his predecessor.

By obliging the feudal lords to take up residence in the capital a social hierarchy developed within the aristocracy of the five great clans that mirrored the geography of the city growing up around a large hill. At the top of the hill Shuri-jo, the kings fortified palace, commanded panoramic views of the local lands, approaches and waterways. Around it, forming a perimeter to the palace, were the large villas of those families connected to the crown by blood, princes and lords, nobles and barons whose allegiance could all be relied upon in times of conflict. Further down the hill the harbour district of Naha became a hub of trade and commerce. It was neighboured by Kumemura, a 12th century settlement populated by Chinese aristocracy tasked with enriching art, politics and court culture.

Finally, the former fishing community of Tomari became an industrious district and home to those lords whose allegiance to the Crown under pressure might be less forthcoming, and who's ancestors were once rivals to the ruling lines during the Three Kingdom Period.

This social prejudice has been noted several times. Kafu Kojo of Koju-ryu once said "The Shizoku of the Tomari region were considered the lowest ranked. They were warehouse watchmen and security guards"

George Kerr, author of *Okinawa - History of an Island People* further highlighted the prestige of being associated with a 'Shuri family' when he wrote:

'On this preeminence of Shuri families and the automatic privileges which residence of Shuri conferred, is based a unique social prestige which persists into the second half of the 20th century.'

'... Whenever Ryukyuans assemble for the first time, in Ryukyu, in Tokyo or in Okinawan communities overseas, it is quickly established whether a man has been born in Shuri, educated in Shuri, or has married a woman of Shuri in that order of important precedence.'

Throughout human history such hierarchal thought patterns as these are first consciously formed by elites to unite and strengthen groups of people but they do so by dividing communities with bigotry. These prejudices, which can manifest as cultural, class or racial expressions usually become ingrained subconsciously and passed down through successive generations; it often takes several generations worth of conscious effort, patience and understanding to dissolve them.

The next day I had arranged to meet another sensei, one who definitely accepted that swords existed in the Ryukyu Kingdom because he taught one of the last remaining Te styles to survive into the 21st century. Mr Takamiyagi of Motobu Udundi. Perhaps he would know how to find Higa sensei too.

14
Sipping Te
'Motobu Udundi, Naminoue
& the Bugeikan'

The arrangement was to meet Takamiyagi at 6:30pm on Naminoue beach; a small sandy beach situated beneath a busy bridge linking Tomari to Naha.

Years ago the beach at Naminoue was a meeting point for Motobu Choyu's 'Tode Research Group'. The group comprised of a gathering of martial artists from various styles of karate and kobudo training together and nourishing their martial arts in a general sense, under a common cause.

Born in 1867 Motobu Choyu was the 11th heir of the Motobu clan's secret 'Te' and began his training from an early age under his father. Later he enriched his training by receiving instruction from teachers visiting the Motobu residence such as Sokon Matsumura, the Kings bodyguard and Itosu his scribe. Across town he studied Tomari-te at the home of Matsumora Kosaku. It is said that at the time there was no one more knowledgable in Okinawan martial arts than Motobu Choyu.

When the Ryukyu Kingdom was officially dissolved into the modern Japanese Empire the tradition of passing the family Te onto the King became obsolete and Choyu's own sons lacked the interest to learn what was then considered an outdated trend. They needed to go and find work and moved to the mainland. Instead it would be the research group's tea-boy who would go on to become the successor to the longest traceable lineage of martial arts on Okinawa. His name was Uehara Seikichi.

The young Uehara quickly showed great promise and vowed to his teacher that one day he'd restore the tradition back to the Motobu family line. A promise he completed in his ninety-ninth year by meeting with the grandson of Choyu now living in Japan.

After the Second World War Uehara taught martial arts and called his style Motobu Udundi out of respect for his life-long master Choyu. Udundi literally means 'martial art of the Udun' a noble rank assigned to the Motobu clan which denoted their connection to the royal bloodline. For this reason Motobu Udundi is sometimes referred to as 'Palace Hand'.

Takamiyagi was a later student of Uehara, who had died in 2004 aged one hundred, so meeting him was something I was looking forward to that evening. Returning from a jog, I showered and walked the short distance from the hostel to Naminoue to meet Mr Takamiyagi and our 'middle man' Joe.

"Joel's come from England to train in Udundi. He's a former student of Mark Bishop." Joe was half Okinawan, half American and worked on one of the military bases. I frowned a little at the association with Mark because firstly, I hadn't told Joe my connection with him, he'd learnt that elsewhere, and secondly I was really here on my own efforts. Besides, Takamiyagi didn't really seem to know who Mark was anyway, he'd never met him.

In his more recent works Mark had written critically of Higa Seitoku and what he deemed his 'quasi religious activities'. Rumours on the grapevine also suggested that the frankness of *Okinawan Karate* had also snubbed a few teachers and groups on the island too. Another persistent rumour, albeit a dubious one, was that the book plagiarised a private text on Okinawan karate styles compiled by a teacher of the Uechi-ryu school years earlier. It didn't. However, without knowing the ins and outs of Mark's interactions on the island I wanted to keep my association with him on the quiet until I could gauge things better. Ultimately I wanted teachers to take me at face value based on my own flaws and merits.

I could never fully understand whether Joe trained with Takamiyagi sensei or was just a helpful 'go between' when people like me turned up out of the blue. Takamiyagi's English was certainly good enough that Joe wasn't going to be needed for translation so instead he drove us around for a few hours as we popped into various karate and kobudo dojos unannounced. It always started something like this:

"So Joel, you want to see some kobudo while you're here on the island?"

"Sure." I replied "That could be good."

"OKAY, LETS GO!" Takamiyagi sensei worked in some capacity on the military bases, possibly as a translator, where he seemed to have picked up a certain Americanised enthusiasm which didn't quite match the image in mind of a senior Okinawan martial arts teacher.

Fifteen minutes later we'd pulled up outside a small dojo with a few trainees working out in brown *dogi's*.

"Is it okay for us to just turn up like this?" I enquired.

"It's fine, this is the way it is here." Takamiyagi was assuring me as we nodded a bow and entered a kobudo session halfway through.

The elderly sensei at the front of the class graciously gestured to some seats and continued counting in a monotonous rhythm as his group of trainees performed their *bo* kata one movement at a time. Then *tonfa*, *nunchaku* and *sai* in similar fashion. At one point Takamiyagi's mobile phone rang and without apology he answered it and had a conversation while the group sweated it out in the humid evening heat. But it was alright, "things are different here Okinawans are more laid back than the mainland." However I did note that when the class finished the three of us were left awkwardly waiting around because the teacher had disappeared out the backdoor never to return. A quiet protest perhaps?

Back in the car, cruising around Naha for our next victim, I mean dojo, to drop in on Takamiyagi made a few phone calls and then announced "You wanna meet Higa sensei whilst you're here in Okinawa?"

"Yes I would, that's really why I've come actually." There was a slight hesitation in my response. A hesitation that was quietly dreading Takamiyagi's fast trending catchphrase so I added, "But all in good time, there's no rush."

"OKAY, LETS GO! - He's not far from here."

Suddenly everything seemed rushed. I wasn't expecting to meet Higa sensei that evening, not without preparation and some token gift of introduction. I was also panicking a little because I didn't fully know the details surrounding Mark's departure from the Bugeikan almost twenty years earlier although I knew it revolved around a disagreement with Higa's father, Seitoku.

Despite my efforts it seemed a karmic ghost was riding on my shoulders whether I liked it or not, so tactfully I tried to explain my hesitations.

I felt bad about playing down my relationship with Mark, after all I had spent a good part of the previous year living with him and I really enjoyed the time and relationship we had. But on another level he had always dissuaded me from travelling to Okinawa claiming "all the real masters are gone now. And you'd probably end up wasting a lot of money." But this was something I felt destined to do, I needed to meet Mr Higa myself, I needed to feel his technique and I needed to come to my own conclusions.

"SURE THING JOEL! Don't worry about it, I'll introduce you to Mr Higa, but I can't say whether he will teach you anything - his mother said he doesn't teach anyone anymore."

"Who is Higa sensei? I'm sure I've heard of him." Joe now glanced sideways as he drove down the street. "Doesn't he have some kind of religious thing going on? I'm sure I saw him at a festival one year all dressed in white doing some crazy stuff."

"Yes. That was him." Takamiyagi's response carried a curt, sceptic tone and I quietly grinned on the backseat. Why do people get so jittery about such things?

As the car turned into the small backstreet I smiled again. We were now passing the exact point where I had had those 'tingling' sensations the night before. It turned out I'd been standing right outside Higa's home all along but didn't know which side of the street it was on.

Takamiyagi instructed Joe to go and park up further ahead which seemed a little odd and felt like a subtle tactic being played as we then entered the house without him and made our way upstairs to a large room with over sixty straw tatami.

There was an intensity in the air that made me feel electric and as I paused in the doorway looking in, Mr Higa was dressed in his white kimono and *haori* jacket. Takamiyagi strode in and I followed at a distant while he began his introduction. Even I could translate it: "This is Joel Reeves, he is a student of MARK BISHOP, from England."

"Mark Bishop?" Higa repeated in near disbelief.

Then the conversation came to describing who Mark was for Takamiyagi's benefit, because although he'd clearly heard the name before he couldn't be sure if he'd ever met him. This was cleared up by Higa sensei simply waving his hands in the air in festival style whilst mimicking the catchphrase "*Yasui Bindai!*", 'It's Cheap!' It seems that Mark's claim to fame on Okinawa was the time he appeared in an advert for an American styled kitchen outlet. To lend a unique memetic quality to the commercial he inspiringly came up with the '*Yasui Bindai*' phrase whilst performing the *kachashi* hand movement of Okinawan dances. Takamiyagi grinned a knowing grin and mimicked the phrase and gesture back with exaggerated form.

Taking a deep breath I nodded and, for a moment that seemed to last an eternity, Higa and I simply looked at each other in silence while Takamiyagi's voice became a rambling background murmur. After a while I nodded again, quietly stepped back and made a bow to the shrine area where a picture of Bugei-no-Kami, the god of martial arts, painted by Higa's father was on display and drawing me in.

"OKAY? Joel!" coming out of a strange reverie, in which all the training and experiences of my life had brought me to this one moment in time, the enquirer's voice seemed muffled and dull. It was Takamiyagi.

"We're going now."

Like waking from a day dream I bowed to Mr Higa, and found myself retreating a few steps backwards. Not through some overt display of reverence but because my instinct was telling me that I didn't want to turn my back and be within striking range of this master; even though he was then seventy-four years old and standing at least fifteen feet away from me he had an aura of intensity that kept me on high alert. Not in a negative way, but nonetheless I wasn't taking any chances.

Leaving the large room we went downstairs to the front door where Joe was waiting outside.

"I didn't know where you two had gone. Did you meet him?"

"Yes. He wants you to come back Thursday evening at 6pm. He'll grant you one lesson. I'll come with you." Takamiyagi glanced back over his shoulder as we got back in the car and drove down into town.

"So he does teach then?" Joe was inquisitively asking, seeming a little disappointed to have not come up to the room with us.

"Not really. But he'll give him a lesson."

We drove on to a fast food restaurant close to Naminoue and stopped for a drink. Joe was still asking Takamiyagi about the meeting who mostly conversed in Japanese broken with bits of English for my benefit. I got the distinct impression that Takamiyagi didn't really approve of Higa's 'spiritual' approach. When we were leaving, a congregation of sorts had already started gathering in the room and there was a distinct 'religious' vibe starting to fill the place as mostly middle-aged women came in and chatted quietly to one another.

"It's not quite ancestor worship, but more his own version of it." Takamiyagi sipped on the straw of his soda as Joe glanced to me.

"And what about you? Did he talk to you? What did he say?"

"HA! He's come all the way from England just to meet him and he didn't even say one word. Not one word!" This notion seemed to entertain Takamiyagi immensely because he laughed an incredulous laugh to which I simply shrugged and responded in all seriousness. "Oh we didn't talk Joe, but we said plenty and understood each other perfectly."

Dropping me back at the hostel I bid them both goodnight and thanked them for showing me around. I enjoyed Takamiyagi's company, he was fun to be around and didn't seem to mind door-stopping teachers although it probably wasn't really the right protocol. Maybe the Okinawans are more relaxed than teachers on the mainland, or maybe Takamiyagi's senior age went some way to breaking down those kind of social barriers.

Tomorrow I'd catch a bus twenty miles north to Koza where Takamiyagi has a dojo and will introduce me to some other teachers of the Motobu Udundi style. An excited energy was coursing through my body and I headed in to have a meal and go to bed.

As it happens I couldn't get to sleep that night on the count of a new guest in the room snoring so deeply it seemed to shake the whole building. Periodically me and one other guest would try to kick his bunk and stir him from his drunken slumber but to no avail, so I got up, slipped outside and went for a walk.

There is a certain sense of insomnia that always accompanies my visits to Japan. More than jet-lag it's something I can't quite describe, like I'm in another world and by coming out at night you get to explore a different side of things without the hustle and bustle of daytime commuters.

In the park adjoining Namninoue there were the homeless living in makeshift shelters or sleeping rough on benches beneath the clear night sky. Most people turn away from the homeless, trying their hardest not to not see them. That for me is the real 'problem' of homelessness; the one where those who live in warm homes and sleep in comfortable beds look away from the tramp through a sense of fear. Not necessarily fear of the 'homeless person' themselves but perhaps a fear of 'becoming' them.

Heading further into town I walked towards a quieter Koksai Dori. No pretty girls at this time, no cartoon-like music or even the hum of the monorail; Naha was sleeping. But a nightmare was forming.

A little after 3am I was drawn by the buzzing sound of a motorbike performing donuts in the centre of what in daytime hours would be a busy intersection. A police car with its siren on parked to one side looked on whilst waiting for backup to arrive. I stopped by the pedestrian crossing watching rider and pillion tease and coax the police with their display of civil disobedience. All the while I obediently waited for the flashing green man to give me permission to cross the otherwise empty street.

The bikers were no real threat, they rode an old style military bike and wore old-style army helmets with painted skulls upon them. A large arial waved from the back of the bike like those on model radio controlled cars. The whole scene seemed a little out of place here but the police just sat watching, as did the few drivers in the cars now missing their green 'go' lights as traffic signals phased red to green and back again. The bikers were travelling so slow even I could've rushed into the road and dragged them off, but of course I just watched. Being Japan I suspect I'd have been in more trouble for just crossing without the green man.

Minutes later another police car arrived, then a third and fourth, all having appeared from different directions. The first pulled forward but it didn't attempt to block the bikers path, instead it gave chase at 10mph going round and round like a little toy. Another joined in. Part of me felt like I must be dreaming but I wasn't. Eventually, as the bikers collected a fifth police car, they opened up the throttle, pulled a wheelie and tore off southbound down route 58 with a fanfare of sirens in hot pursuit. Except it wasn't really a 'hot' pursuit because it seemed as though the speed of the police cars were restricted to a manufacturers default. So instead they adopted a perfect chevron formation behind the bike racing away.

It was yet another demonstration of Japanese non-confrontation. As far as the police were concerned no-one had been hurt, the riders had had their fun and were now being escorted out of the town centre.

Quiet descended like a blanket. Naha was sleeping and the only noticeable movement was the changing sequences of traffic lights.

Further ahead, down the back streets of Koksai Dori the buzz of mopeds whizzed about in the shadows like so many wasps. It's hard to tell whether it was safe to be out or not. I suspect it was but there was a tension in the air so I turned back.

Heading to Naminoue, with the cool sand underfoot slipping through my toes, I sat for a while watching moonlit waves lap upon the shore. Quietly, with heavy eyes, I pulled my hood up, laid upon a grassy verge and drifted to sleep.

This island breathed a history that seemed alive.

15
Koza

"In Te the only way to learn a technique is to feel it"

Koza, or 'Okinawa City' is a 20km bus ride north of Naha and doesn't share the capitals' tourist-like charm on the count of it being so close to a large US airbase. Many of the small businesses along the streets appeared closed down and despite being a thoroughfare for traffic travelling north and south there was a certain gritty, run down feeling to the area.

In late December of 1970 Koza was the scene of a large-scale anti American riot when two US marines driving under influence knocked down an Okinawan civilian crossing the street. No serious injury was incurred but a number of taxi drivers who had witnessed the event started to antagonise the marines and surrounded their vehicle.

Incidents like these always left a bitter taste because the US personnel could never be prosecuted under local law, even if they were off duty and committed crimes in civilian areas. Tensions were running particularly high because a few months earlier a housewife from Itoman had been killed in a similar hit and run incident from which the marines involved were acquitted at court-martial.

In the Koza incident a crowd started to form with angry chants of "Yankee go home" and "no more acquittals". The situation was made worst when a second American vehicle arriving on scene struck another civilian. The crowd swelled throwing rocks and taunts. Before the end seven hundred MPs were deployed against a crowd of five thousand. When tear gas was used the crowd ran amok throwing petrol bombs, turning over cars, smashing American property and breaking through the perimeter fence of the nearby airbase where they torched several buildings.

The Koza Riot was the release valve of an enforced American occupation that had been in place since the close of WWII. In 1972 political control of the island was handed to Japan, despite a strong desire for independence from the islanders. Since that time incidents to date involving US personnel against civilians include gang rapes, bar fights and aircraft crashes in public areas. Not to mention the illegal storing and transporting of chemical and nuclear weapons on the bases. At the time of writing there is ongoing resistance for plans to build a new airbase in the north of the island which will have devastating consequences to already endangered wildlife and their natural habitat including the Okinawan Dugong. These extremely rare and gentle sea dwelling creatures, likened to a 'sea cow', are at a critical juncture with less than fifteen remaining at the current time of writing. Their primary habitat is the site of the new US Air Base.

The ongoing problems of US occupation are not going to disappear anytime soon. Since the close of WWII the island has played a strategic role for US operations in Korea and Vietnam and it will remain America's foothold in the Pacific Theatre for any potential conflicts of the future.

To put the Okinawan side of the argument into perspective, despite representing only 1% of Japanese land, Okinawa Island houses 75% of the US military bases in Japan, with nearly 25,000 US personnel and their families stationed there which is almost equal to a quarter of the domestic population.

Yet public opinion over the US presence is split. For many, the bases provide a source of income through land rentals and employment. Presumably people like Takamiyagi. For others there is strong contention about the social influences such as noise, pollution and the threat to wildlife caused by the bases.

Takamiyagi's dojo was situated above an old shop that looked out over the sprawling urban area in two directions. It was modest but functional with a tatami floor, hanging punchbag and various sticks, bokkens and sparring equipment lining the walls.

He began his session with a series of natural exercises to encourage the relaxation and suppleness required for Udundi training. Then came the basic footwork, punching, striking and kicking drills that form a sort of 'karate-like' aspect to the style. Takimiyagi has done a great deal to try and 'systemise' the Motobu Udundi he learnt from Uehara, which, compared with karate in a general sense, is significantly more liberated in its approach to training and lacks the ordered structure of a syllabus.

When it came to kicking, Takamiyagi would shake his head in disapproval at my attempts with a simple statement.

"No." Frustratingly he would offer no more guidance on what he wanted to see but just laughed saying it wasn't correct. I already knew what the issue was though. When he held a padded shield for me to kick he nodded approvingly.

"Yes! That's it!" But without the target he would shake his head no again. It seemed it was the fact I wasn't allowing my knee to hyper extend whilst kicking the air. A silly habit from my early karate years and one I wasn't about to re-adopt. Training against the air is different to striking a target, whether moving or stationary, so you must always look after your joints and adjust martial technique accordingly.

In comparison to karate kicks those of Te are performed with a hop type shuffle and delivered from the front leg with the heel lifted on the supporting foot. Although fast, it tends to 'tread' forward into the target rather than 'snapping' as is taught in karate.

After the basics had been thoroughly worked we switched pace and followed the movements of Uehara via a small television performing the dance '*Hamchidori*'. The choreography of the movements were not ingrained in to Takamiyagi's mind and so several times we got the 'mirroring' wrong at which point we'd have to hurriedly catch up as Uehara gracefully twirled and glided through the steps.

Hamachidori isn't one of the classical Court Dances through which Te technique had been secretly codified in the 18th century but it did have all the fundamental movements for beginners to more easily learn from. Floating footwork, posture, rhythm and the *kachashi* hand movements that comprise of *ogami-te*, *konari-te* and *oshi-te*, rising, turning and pushing hand; the central techniques of Motobu Udundi's unique grappling method called *tuiti*

When the session ended we drove off to visit a friend studying Ryukyuan history and further discussed Motobu Udundi and it's connection with *kumiodori* dance.

In the later part of his life Uehara Seikichi had devoted much time to exploring this relationship and performed a number of public demonstrations revealing the subtle, yet highly effective, grappling techniques found within their graceful movements.

Unlike the more vibrant folk dances performed at village festivals, which share similarities to karate and kobudo, the court dances are slow and sedate with an appearance closer to Tai Chi. The hand gestures in both genre's are universal but whereas in folk dance the movements are often grand and expressive, in court style they are subtle and performed in a meditative state with centred movement.

The oldest collection of these dances are categorised as '*Onna Odori*', the 'Women's Dances' and were performed to visiting Chinese envoys during the Ryukyu Kingdom era by senior males of the Shuri aristocracy.

In these performances, dexterity, balance and elegance are the signs of a skilled exponent. With footwork reminiscent of

Japanese Noh Theatre the performer appears to be 'floating on clouds' while the arms are held in a soft arc similar to that of western ballet. The *Onna-odori* themes convey tales of love and its impermanence; lost, found and hopeless, reflected in the dream-like triangular gaze of the performer. These dances were never seen outside of Shuri Palace which is partly why 'Te' technique slipped from common knowledge when karate 'styles' first began to emerge in the early 1900's.

Occasionally a dancer added deeper meaning to their movements through the employment of a simple prop such as the parasol, weavers spool or willow sprig. With martial insight it is apparent that such props, when replaced with classical weapons like sword, glaive and spike and shield, describe combative techniques with perfect form that mirror the unique entry strategies of Te.

The prevailing theory then is that traditional Okinawan dances such as *Muto*, *Kashiki* and *Yanajii* amount to a collection of sorts, of Te kata and Uehara Seikichi was instrumental in unlocking this aspect of Motobu Udundi.

That evening I stayed at Takamiyagi's home with a selection of texts on Uehara for bedtime reading. Although it is not widely known, he influenced a far greater number of modern karate and kobudo teachers than is realised. His early training with Choyu Motobu consisted mostly of a free-style *kumite* called *jissen*, where only the roles of attacker and defender are pre-defined. During this time period almost all other *bujin* of note on Okinawa were teaching kata.

Like my training with Mark, attacks in *jissen* training were un-determined and forced you to read the subtle clues in an opponent's posture and approach. It wasn't until several generations later that karate teachers started to introduce *kumite* into their styles at all, and even then it was in a pre-arranged fashion with block then strike combinations.

During the 1960's Uehara began teaching *tuiti* grappling, to a gathering of senior *bujin* including Higa Seitoku who openly said that at that time 'no one in Okinawan martial arts understood the practice of *tuiti* other than Uehara'. And he would know. Higa had trained privately to a senior level with many of the last old-school teachers.

The following morning I woke early, rolled away my futon and performed some light stretches while I waited to hear Takamiyagi sensei say "OKAY LET'S GO!" The plan was to head to the beach for some training.

I'd heard about Uehara's morning beach sessions before. Since his passing in 2004 they had been continued by a senior long-term student named Mrs Arasaki. Takamiyagi was taking me to train with them now although it seemed that was to be something of a problem.

Perhaps it was another unannounced 'drop in' because as we arrived the group prematurely wrapped things up and headed back to their cars.

Mature and beautiful in her natural demeanour Arasaki sensei had a certain sternness to her voice that seemed to grow in intensity as Takamiyagi conversed with her. Being the target of several sideways glances I gave up on trying to introduce myself and kept back. Her senior student shared an awkward shrug with his eyes while he also fidgeted uncomfortably to one side.

It would be wrong to say I understood all that was said but the general impression was that I wasn't welcome and Takamiyagi sensei was getting his ear chewed for bringing me along. It wasn't necessarily a personal thing against me, at least I don't think so, but since Uehara's death, the successorship of the Udundi style had been officially passed to the now ageing nephew of Choyu Motobu and the style was quickly becoming stifled by hierarchal politics from the honbu dojo in Japan. Motobu Udundi was becoming a closed system and entrance to training needed to come through approved recommendations. I didn't have one.

The honcho of the Motobu Ryu Udundi style is presently Chosei Motobu, a grandson to Choyo Motobu and the third son of Chokki Motobu who is more known in karate circles for his no-nonsense approach to fighting.

Chosei, who is now ninety, holds both his father's karate and the Motobu Te system of his ancestors. However, perhaps due to living on the mainland all his life, his thought patterns seem to favour their approach of forming tightly regulated organisations with a strict grading structure and hierarchy. All in the interest of preserving 'purest' ideas of style and lineage of course. Though I suspect financial gain plays some small part too.

In 2012, a couple of years after I returned from Okinawa, the official Motobu Ryu website went all out in a ranting dialogue to clarify in no uncertain terms just 'who' they recognise as legitimate instructors of the style. In Japan there are thirteen. In Okinawa there is only one; Mrs Arasaki. This seems incredulous considering that Uehara spent no significant time teaching on the mainland. Yet despite this there are a considerable number of sensei on Okinawa who spent long periods of time, decades in fact, training directly under him. Some were granted 6th-10th dan ranks including Takamiyagi, his teacher Shian Toma, Takao Miyagi, Akamine sensei in Naha and Arakawa sensei in Okinawa City. Higa Kiyohiko himself holds a *hanshi* grade awarded directly from Uehara. Those are just the one's I came to know about. Uehara also had a son, Takeshi who continues to teach in Naha between running a successful dentist practice.

These teachers however seem to have become excommunicated from the newly formed *honbu*. To quote the official Motobu-ryu website in their own prose:

'There were instances throughout history when an instructor was removed from the organization by the soke [grandmaster], having their standing and credentials cancelled, no longer to represent the art. These decisions were exclusively made by the soke, whether in Motobu Udundi by Uehara Seikichi Sensei before he passed the art of Motobu Udundi back to the Motobu Family (in 2003) or by Motobu Chosei Soke.'

Perhaps it wasn't so much that the Okinawan teachers were being excluded by Chosei but rather they themselves were refraining from coming under his banner? The Okinawans are a proud people and there isn't a more 'patriotic' martial art representative of Ryukyu culture than Udundi.

Although nothing was ever said to me during my time in Koza it was clear that the politics of Motobu-ryu were driving a sizeable wedge between those teachers on the mainland who held 'legitimate rank' and those on the island with years of 'legitimate training'. People will have to decide for themselves where the true Te rests.

Or maybe Uehara left a subtle clue for future generations just like Funakoshi did with his karate. During one of his last recorded interviews Uehara stated:

'The most important thing for young trainees is to find a good teacher. Style is not important. Find a good teacher and you can't go wrong.'

Over a McDonalds-esque breakfast Takamiyagi appeared a little dejected by the mornings events. We had of course just witnessed another case of Ryukyuan non-confrontational diplomacy. We wanted to train. They didn't want to train with us, so they left. Takamiyagi's frustration came from wanting to forge ahead with teaching Udundi as it had been passed to him by his teacher. The 'official' line from Japan however was to 'hold on' and let things settle.

"I'm seventy-three years old! I don't have time to 'hold on!'" He vented as we wallowed in the closed-minded attitude that was plaguing Motobu-ryu. His teacher before him, Shian Toma had only recently died following the return trip from teaching in the States and for me Takamiyagi appeared to carry weight over this.

I suggested there were enough teachers on Okinawa to form their own group. On a karmic level Uehara had already absolved himself of any debt to his teacher when he returned the 'successorship' of the style back into the Motobu family, as per his wishes. Surely now it was up to Uehara's students how they proceeded with the knowledge he had shared with them?

To break the curse of the moment I asked Takamiyagi about whether he considered Te a unique art-form separate from karate and kobudo. It was a question that had been lingering in my mind for a while and seeing as he had come from a background in karate I was interested to hear his response.

"In Motobu Udundi the term 'Te' implies a 'method' or 'technique'; as in *'kashin-te'*, 'battle-hands' and *'tui-ti'*, 'grappling hands'. As well as *konari-te*, *ogami-te* etcetera. Te is not really a distinct system of it's own. I think when people speak of Te like that then they are really talking about *tuiti*.".

Pushing away the plastic tray and discarded food wrappers Takamiyagi shook off the sombre atmosphere and announced.
"So you wanna see some more kobudo?"
"Sure!" I smiled.
"OKAY LETS GO!

*

Entering through a side door we stepped onto the polished wooden floor of Mr Uchina's kobudo and dance dojo.

Uchina sensei teaches kobudo and Udundi while his wife teaches traditional Okinawan dance. I don't know if he had been given prior notice of our arrival or not but he welcomed us in and generously arranged a demonstration for my benefit. The performers were a troupe of teenage girls who were happy for me to film them as they performed several dances armed with *nunchaku*, *sai* and *eku*, the traditional Okinawan 'oar' and probably one of the oldest weapons of Te.

The girls' movements were crisp and disciplined yet carried a rhythmic fluidness that was thoroughly captivating. Despite their age it was clear they had an understanding of how to wield each weapon and their grips and footwork revealed knowledge of Te as well. The girls also enjoyed a certain level of fame, for throughout the year they perform demonstrations such as the one I was privy to at festivals and functions all over the island.

Glancing along the portraits of masters overseeing training at the dojo was one of Uehara Seikichi looking down with his genial, approving smile. Although I never witnessed Mr Uchina perform a single technique I knew enough, based upon the quality of his young students, that I would have liked to train there during my stay were it not for the long commute from Naha.

Leaving Mr Uchina and the dancing girls behind we drove off to visit another former student of Uehara's, in the area. Mr Arakawa.

The term 'master' is not one I freely assign to many individuals but for Mr Arakawa it fits well. his dojo was a small, narrow room above an apartment somewhere. Whereas at the Uchina dojo I was privileged to witness a demonstration of technique, here I was requested to give one.

For quarter of an hour Arakawa and his senior student put me through my paces as I demonstrated the fundamental footwork, punching and kicking drills of the Udundi style. It was a grading of sorts. A way of gauging not only the quality of my technique but the effort I was willing to put in too. And the effort paid off. My reward was that Arakawa sensei granted me a lesson.

Wearing a pair of shorts and a short sleeve shirt he signalled for me to grab him however I pleased. By his wrists, the lapels or collar, it didn't matter. No sooner had I entered I found myself flung down one end of the dojo. Space was so tight that several times I had to re-throw myself into a second roll just to avoid smashing into the walls.

Each time I tried to grab him it felt as though he wasn't really there at all; as if I were simply holding a cotton shirt up to the wind. There was no 'push, pull' sensation which would normally follow grabbing someone. No anchoring or sense of weight at all. It really was like holding up an empty shirt.

Within this hold, using the subtlest of body movements, Arakawa would not only break my balance but my grip too - now I was grabbed by him and felt like a rag as he tossed me around.

It was a curious sensation and picking myself from the ground over and over again I kept coming back to feel more. In Te the only way to learn a technique is to feel it.

For the next hour I practised various techniques like this with his student. In comparison to his teacher his technique was heavy, but mine was even cruder. For a while it became a frustrating experience as we applied force where really we should've been using technique. It felt as though he had something to prove and all I wanted was to feel Arakawa's technique some more. Of course it wasn't like that really, his student and I were bonding, albeit with a sense of machismo, and I suspect he was hoping I'd stay around in Koza to be his training partner for a while.

"How long will you be here? Where are you staying? What days can you train?"

Wiping the sweat from our red flushed faces we grinned and chatted a while as Takamiyagi told Arakawa sensei of my intention to train with Higa Kiyohiko. With a subtle raise of the brow Arakaki enquired how it came to be that I would train with Higa, on the count that he no longer accepted students. For this of course Takamiyagi brought up my connection to Mark Bishop, via a reference to the '*Yasui Bindai*' commercial of yesteryear which prompted Arakaki sensei to grin nosltalgicly . Clearly a testament to the persuasiveness of TV commercials if ever one were needed.

With the late afternoon sun causing the streets outside to shimmer in a haze of heat we eventually said our goodbyes and headed off in the car. My t-shirt and training bottoms were pulled and torn from training but there was suddenly no time to get changed as Takamiyagi hurriedly dropped me at a bus stop.

"I've had a call from my wife and need to go home. You'll have to go to Higa on your own this evening. On Monday you should come back here and look to find somewhere to stay so you can train with us." Checking his watch he added "You'd better hurry, you've just over an hour and a half."

And that was the last time I saw Takamiyagi or any of the other's from Koza. It had been a packed few days and a real eye-opener that will remain in my thoughts for years to come, but ultimately I was here to learn from Higa sensei, and although I would have loved to train back in Koza, one thing led to another.

An hour and a half was barely enough time at all to get to the Bugeikan. Arriving in Tomari I ran back to the hostel, borrowed a bicycle and raced into town to catch the monorail to Gibo. All in the nick of time.

I was about to meet another master.

16
Kaminchu

"Does your friend have his own religion too?"

In a village east of Shuri a young woman helps an ageing neighbour with his house chores and meals. She is not his granddaughter, he is no relative at all, but he is alone and she helps him nonetheless.

"I've met a new friend from England." She tells him whilst tidying away after lunch. "He is training in *bujutsu*."

"Oh?" He responds. "Where is he training? Naha?"

"Hai. His sensei's name is Higa-san, Higa Kiyohiko."

"Higa sensei!" He exclaims "I know him." With a playful glint in his eye he leans forward and touches her arm.

"He has his own religion you know. Does your friend have his own religion too?" With a reprimanding smile she shakes her head and asks how it is he knows about Higa sensei.

"School. He was always very special. Could do special things. Even from an early age he excelled in karate and his *bojutsu* was of the expert level too. It might not mean much to you but his teacher was Masami Chinen of Yamane-ryu. Higa-sensei inherited his style." He smiled and went outside to inspect some flowers in the sunny garden.

"His father taught *bujutsu* too. His name was Higa Seitoku. One day I heard a story that he awoke from a dream in which he envisioned a Sage performing a mystical martial art. It was different than any karate style he'd seen before. In the middle of the night he went to his son's bedroom, who was already *nidan* in karate. 'Wake up!' he told him. 'Put your karate *gi* on and meet me downstairs in the dojo.' Placing a sword in his son's hands he told him "Now, attack me as if you mean to kill me. Do it!" "But father?" His son protested. "DO IT! ..."'

Squatting down with child-like innocence she listened wide-eyed as the neighbour re-told the story of Higa sensei and his special martial art. '"He says it's inspired by the *kami*. It's called Shin Do Ryu."'

This is how stories of the martial arts have been passed down on Okinawa since time immemorial. It was a year later when my friend first shared it with me and when she did she re-told it with all the heart of a story-teller entertaining a child.

*

Slipping my shoes off in the doorway I made my way upstairs for my lesson with Higa sensei.

Normally, in my experience, when a sensei meets a potential trainee he will not engage him in *kumite* and certainly not in front of students. It could be risky. But then, Higa is no ordinary sensei.

When I arrived that evening one other was present. Hirokazu Isyado. Perhaps some twenty years my senior Isyado had a serious face and sturdy build. When I met him he was tying a *tenugui* towel about his head. Isyado had trained directly under Higa Seitoku for forty years and since the master's death he'd continued under his son Kiyohiko. The back of Isyado's worn white gi had the kanji for "Shin Do Ryu" brushed upon its canvas in thick black ink. 'Way of the Gods'.

With a measuring nod he bowed and led me into basic training with a series of punches and kicks. The style was similar to that practised in the Motobu dojos but differed slightly. At the Bugeikan the footwork was more liberated and although it might at first appear sloppy to an onlooker it is in fact more reflective of technique against a live opponent. That is, they feel more fluid and practical. The second discernible feature is the extensive range of kicks. Whereas Motobu Udundi taught just one, the Bugeikan had several including front, side, crescent, reverse and back.

With the *kihon* basics covered, for there are no blocks in either Motobu Udundi or at the Bugeikan, Isyado had seen enough and Higa sensei arrived.

There was no time wasted. With a smile and a nod he stood before me dressed in his white kimono, opened his arms and issued a simple command. "Attack."

For me it had become the mark of a true master and the last of three traits by which I personally ranked a teacher worth training under. So many would rather wear you down with a student or two while they watched from the sideline assessing your technique and strategy. Of those who might then grant you an opportunity to 'attack' the majority will say "grab here" or "hit me" as they pat their belly. To have a tenth dan invite an open attack is both rare and speaks volumes of their confidence. I was having an awakening of a different sorts.

Glancing to Isyado, checking his proximity and position to my side, he nodded and stepped away. Then, with eyes on Higa I assumed a *kamae*, stalked forwards a few paces, and launched a lighting fast triple punch combination to the head. With the subtlest of movements Higa slipped the attack at the final moment, his loose sleeves and flowing *hakama* swished about me and I was dropped painfully to the tatami with a foot locking my leg and a twisted arm pinning my shoulder. With a flick of the wrist and a smile he thrust me away into a forward roll and I sprung back to my feet.

The range had opened up so for my second attack I rushed forward feigning a kick to the chest and then leaping the gap with a one, two head shot. Again he slipped aside, jabbed his fingers into my ribs and seized the lapel of my gi to cast me down to the tatami. Had I not known to roll using Te's unique *ukemi* rolling techniques I would have landed awkwardly with a jolted neck for sure.

I was determined to hit Higa but not with malice nor the frustrated anger that came out with Mark two years earlier. My technique and attitude had changed since those days. I'd like to think it'd matured.

Before arriving in Okinawa a 'keyboard warrior' had posted video clips online of Higa demonstrating at a Shuri festival from the late nineties. The footage was labeled as an example of 'distant' or 'no touch' knockouts and cast dubious suspicion as he appeared to project advancing students away by simply waving his hands in the air.

There was more to it than that, but people's ignorance was only heightened by the editing out of earlier parts of the day's demonstration in which Higa defended against full on attacks both armed and unarmed. What was left was really a light-hearted exercise in sensitivity to 'intrinsic' energy or, *ki*. The group was having fun with it. Playing.

There was no way I had come this far to simply 'allow' Higa to beat me. If I came away from all this with a broken arm or worst I didn't care, I intended to do my best to strike him. Of course in reality his technique was so superb I was at no risk of gaining such injury. Nonetheless I tried my best and held nothing back.

Rolling out of distance from any counter-attack I stood up with eyes narrowed scanning for an opening. Higa was already advancing towards me with arms by his sides and striding confidently. With a racing heart I rapidly drove a fist forward whilst over-arm grabbing at his lapel in an attempt to tackle and throw. In a blink my wrist became trapped in a spiralling swirl and my legs came up behind my head as I was pinned painfully in a lock once more. My punch hadn't even glanced him.

Released, I looked up from my half kneeling position as he walked away. He wasn't reckless enough to turn his back but with a *kiai* to summon my strength I drove out of my half squat with the ball of my foot aimed squarely at his flank. Without so much of a flinch he side stepped into the movement, thrust his palm into my chest and swept my supporting leg away with his footwork.

His eyes flashed a look as he urged me to try again. This was *jissen!*

Heart pounding and sweat streaking my face I exhaled sharply, stood up and raised my fists. Just at that moment Higa lurched with a movement that made me feel as though he was attacking.

Already a little dazed, my limbs felt heavy and the adrenalin was deafening my ears. Moving on auto-pilot I wasn't even aware of what type of attack I was attempting as I rushed forward. Four feet away an accusing finger thrust at my abdomen and I flinched in the final moment. Taking advantage of my error he entered, took my hands, and flung me across five tatami. Without time to roll I managed only to turn mid-air and fall flat on my belly with limbs akimbo. Like a frog falling from the sky. It was all I could do to not be winded.

This was crazy. I hadn't even touched him once. Bringing myself to my feet I went all out to land a blow.

Twelve feet. Ten. Six. Four. Higa remained poised and strode towards me out of time with my advance. His open hands suddenly jabbed the air between us, each one seeming to not only highlight the openings in my guard but strike me too. My body responded as if I'd been struck. It didn't hurt, I hadn't even been touched, but I felt it.

Trying to complete my attack, a double one, two punch and kick, Higa was in range but his movements so fluid we didn't even collide. Being so close I should have been able to blindly grab him in a clinch but when I tried it was like tumbling into an abyss. Again I crashed to the tatami.

Exhausted. Exhilarated. Overwhelmed.

With breathing ragged I got up and launched another attack. My final one. I gave it everything I had left. Higa *kiai'd* sharply and held an open palm towards me. My momentum stopped, body leant backwards and my legs felt like lead. With eyes locked on mine his open hand clenched to a fist and he pulled the air between us.

Propelled forwards I stumbled drunkenly and threw one final punch before collapsing at his feet. It was over. A battle on several fronts. What had just happened I couldn't be sure but I felt utterly spent and drained of all fighting spirit.

Clinging to the mats like a baby I'm aware that Higa knelt by my side resting his palms upon my back. I'm not ashamed to say that tears filled my eyes as I breathed upon the cool straw tatami. Tears of happiness. My mind stopped searching for answers.

People have since asked 'what happened?' and so I try to explain it like this: In the first instance all techniques were physical, Higa avoided my strikes and projected me with regular throws and locks. But then things changed. He seemed to expose and then strike my openings without touch. Maybe it was mental, like hypnosis, or maybe he'd manipulated some invisible connection between us. *Ki*. It felt more than hypnosis though. More tangible. It 'felt' physical.

The final phase was as though his very presence had somehow sapped me of all energy. When he pulled his empty fist close I found myself propelled like a stretched rubber band springing back to its original form.

Laying there, with the application of his hands upon my back, I felt a new warmth rise through my bones and radiate into my muscles. All of these sensations of course occurred on a personal level, whether you or anyone else would experience the same is hard to know. But it would be no exaggeration to say that I felt as though all the stress, worry and anxiety of the past were washed from me. Not just the past few minutes, or even weeks, but years. Maybe even lifetimes?

It strikes me as odd that many in the karate world today doubt the ability of a no-touch knockdown like the one I have just recounted, Yet at the same time many will happily recount the tale of the legendary Bushi Matsumura who, without laying a finger upon the famous karateka Uehara, defeated him in a challenge match at the Kinbu Palace graveyard.

Like me Uehara was no novice to fighting yet he too succumbed to a non-physical attack. It was more than mental because at an advanced level we can rise above the destructive elements of an adrenal rush and 'fight from the void'.

Would such a technique work on a common street mugger? Possibly. However I suspect that even if such an unlikely event were ever to occur even Higa sensei would probably respond in a physical way. Why risk otherwise?

Which begs the question, 'would a no-touch defeat work on someone not 'emotionally' attached to the one performing it?' That is, would Higa's technique work on a student from another school or with no martial arts background at all? Again I have no definitive answer one way or the other. From a personal perspective I went 'all out' to hit him and frustratingly failed at every opportunity. As far as I was aware this one session was the only opportunity I was going to get to train with him. However I also feel that even asking such a question is to miss the point. The purpose of the technique is not so much about fighting but more like a form of bodywork similar to shiatsu. Albeit a more vigorous one.

Pulling my legs up under myself I crawled into a ball and bowed my head. This was a teacher I could really learn something from.

For the final hour of training two more trainees arrived and, with the help of his eldest daughter translating, Higa sensei afforded me a great honour. He didn't accept new students but he invited me to attend his home every evening, except Sundays, where I would receive three hours of personal tuition. On Wednesdays and Fridays my training would be overseen by Isyado.

Kata were prescribed, *Naihanchi* and *Sanchin*, in order to develop my physique and provide a foundation for new techniques. Later would come other forms, *Nidanbu*, *Sanpabu* and weapons kata besides.

During the days I was welcome to train in the dojo alone where I had access to a wide range of weapons under the watchful eyes of Higa Seitoku's portrait and a painting of

153

Bugei-no-Kami. Although most days I would train at Naminoue where I could improve my stances in the waves or practise footwork in the sand.

I felt like the bionic man, about to be rebuilt anew. The responsibility of my basic training was handed over to Isyado who it seemed for many weeks was incapable of smiling and gave me a much needed 'harshness' that quickly elevated my fitness. Speaking no English he taught by rote and drilled me relentlessly the length and breadth of the dojo until my lungs screamed for air and the muscles in my legs passed the stage of trembling fatigue. For the large part this training consisted of kata, footwork, punching, kicking and throws, saving more advanced aspects of Te training to Higa sensei.

*

It's important to reflect on that 'other' aspect of Higa's persona that seems to cause others to avoid him. At the end of each session a congregation of sorts would start to drift into the dojo. Mostly they comprised of women, middle-aged and senior but also husbands too as well as, labourers and a few university students. During this time Higa would adopt a different role, something more akin to that of a priest, a counsellor, a community leader, a medium and a shaman all in one. The correct term is *Kaminchu* - a spiritually connected person.

Not once did I ever feel obliged to stay and partake in the ceremonies that followed but usually I would of my own accord. For me it was important to witness this aspect of Higa's work and it also provided me a rare insight into a part of Okinawan culture most foreigners are unlikely to ever see.

The traditional religion of Okinawa is Ancestors Worship, which really amounts to paying respect to your ancestors. As the 'Original Ancestors' of everyone are in a sense the sea, land and heaven then the practice becomes one of 'respect for nature' too and shares similarities with Japanese Shinto.

The Ryukyu Islands have maintained a distinct form of Ancestors Worship that differs from that of the mainland despite the arrival of Confucianism, Buddhism and Catholicism being introduced over the years. Although that is not to say that Okinawan Ancestors Worship has not been influenced or enriched by these religions in one way or another too. Traditionally, Ancestors Worship has worked in alliance with a *kaminchu*, a person who is able to transcend the realm between this physical world and that of the spirits. Such people, like Higa sensei, can still be found and form an anchor for Okinawans within their local community.

Several colloquial phrases also tell of this interconnected understanding of the physical and spiritual worlds such as "Half a problem is for a doctor and half a *yuta*." A *yuta* being one of the more 'psychically' active of the *kaminchu* class of individuals which also include the former *noro* Royal Priestesses, as well as *ukuri* clan priests or priestess' and the *usagiyā*, individual's specialising in giving prayer.

With the exception of *noro* which were born into their roles as a matter of royal lineage, most other *kaminchu* are individuals who have 'found themselves' following a period of intense introspection, sometimes coming after nothing short of a mental break-down but not always. Returning to daily life such individuals find themselves able to help those suffering from problems mostly caused by trying to live how others want them to, such as parents, peer pressure and social influences from media, rather than being true to their inner nature.

In rare cases, rather than through a traumatic upbringing or breakdown, the *kaminchu* is inspired to pursue a 'heroes journey', leading them away from society for a time to live alone in nature whilst they contend with physical and supernatural hardship. When they return they do so as sensitive's, seer's and healers.

At the Higa household the usual flow of these proceedings has Higa sensei's eldest daughter collect 'prayer requests' from members of the congregation seeking assistance. Perhaps a mother is being troubled in her dreams or worrying about a son studying on the mainland. Many such cases seem to be examples of psychosomatic problems induced by the sufferer's sub-conscious. In such instances Higa sensei mutters a prayer of invocation inviting the 'Original Ancestors' and a number of lesser *kami* spirits, to be in attendance. "Utin, Jichu, Ryūgū... Fodo Myōō... Bishamonten..."

A small tatami mat, approximately two-foot by one, becomes a stage of sorts by which *kami* can be summoned and communicated with to find appeasement or be banished. Although rather than banish, powerful *kaminchu* like Higa will liberate and transform malevolent spirits into a power for good.

Kami are amoral in character. The traditional belief is that they are neither good nor bad, but can manifest as benign or destructive to human interests depending on the treatment they receive. Dreams form perhaps the most traversed bridge between their world and ours and it seems that the *kami* are able to more easily communicate with their intended recipient through the dream-state in which they appear as themselves or send messages via an attendant.

During a *remui* or a 'divine dream' the *kami* will appear either as an Old Sage, a beautiful woman or serpent-like dragon, but in other cases they will send a messenger in the form of animals, birds or boys. Dream interpretation is thus a large factor in the work of the *kaminchu*.

From my observation during these sessions Higa will enter a trance-like state through which he can more easily communicate with the *kami* and find solutions to problems perplexing the dreamer. I suspect that intent plays a large part of the summoning process and that by stimulating either alpha, or possibly theta, brainwave patterns the right frequency to bridge the conscious and subconscious can be facilitated for communication. In contrast to the shamanic practices of South America, which have of late received popular interest in various sub-cultures about the world, all of Higa's work is done through a meditative process, sometimes sedentary and sometimes through free-movement, but always without the use of herbs.

Whatever the mechanics of it all, it was feasible at times to observe the *kami* arrive and enter into conversation with Higa who would intermittently break from trance to ask a question of the sufferer in order to arrive at a resolution. It's all a case of being on the right frequency which advanced martial arts training cultivates.

Ultimately ritual purity on the part of the worshipper is what the *kami* will find most pleasing. For this reason Higa sensei goes about his conduct on a daily basis with propriety and observance to ceremony.

In recent years research into this aspect of Okinawan culture has tried to map the content of such rituals and ceremonies upon models of modern psychology with varying degrees of success. Ultimately the desired outcome of both fields to influence a positive change in the way an individual thinks, approaches a problem or views other family members is the same.

17
A dog named Shen
"They must fight, to know their place"

During my time on Okinawa I would teach yoga and *kiko* some mornings to a group of local hostel workers and bar staff from the neighbourhood down on Naminoue Beach. Other days I would take field trips to castles, museums and sacred groves. Ultimately I was there for the training.

At the hostel I met a new friend. Marcos. He lived on the mainland and had travelled to Okinawa to visit the main dojo of his chosen karate style, Uechi-ryu.

The origins of this style began with one Kanbun Uechi who, in 1897 and aged twenty, travelled to China to study Chinese boxing. Over a few years he learnt herbalism and kung-fu from a master who wandered the countryside gathering, preparing and selling remedies in the small towns and villages along the way. During these excursions Kanbun would perform kata and body hardening exercises at the roadside to wow passerby's into buying their ointments and lotions.

Years later he returned to Okinawa but for a long time refused to teach anyone his kung-fu. Eventually the style passed to his son Kanyei Uechi who constructed a full-time dojo in Futenma and in turn handed the art to his son Kanmei. Uechi-ryu is what is called a 'family style' and today has branch dojo's around the world.

At the core of the system is a version of the *kata Sanchin*, that trademark kata of Goju-ryu in which trainees slither along the floor hissing like snakes whilst slowly burning every ounce of oxygen in their contracting muscles. The Uechi version differs from that of Goju in that the techniques are somewhat lighter, with open hands instead of fists and a breathing method less forced; albeit still unnatural.

The version of Sanchin I was being taught by Isyado differed too. Called '*Shuri-ti Sanchin*', not only to distinguish it from the others but presumably hinting at its place of origin as well, it utilised an upright posture with natural footwork and breathing from the *hara* which becomes less observable as practitioners advance.

The *Naihanchi kata* I was learning differed from the versions practised in other styles too. It incorporated sinking and twisting movements that serve to develop a unique striking method that generates its power from the waist rather than the hips. Once learnt the appearance of the form flows like a a great river, soft and fluid, crashing and wild, then soft again.

Called *Tachimura Naihanchi*, after its progenitor Bushi Tachimura, the applications of the form are multi-layered and carry a certain Chinese flavour. At a rudimentary level they teach a range of boxing skills whilst developing a robust physique, then there are methods of entering and breaking an opponent's balance. At an advanced level the applications reveal a range of subtle grappling and throwing techniques more akin to the *tuiti* of Te.

Working from the outer to the inner, along with the addition of several 'auxiliary' exercises, you come to realise that *Tachimura Naihanchi* is practically a style unto itself.

Both *Sanchin* and *Naihanchi*, are important kata's in Okinawan karate. Generally speaking Okinawan karate styles can be categorised into one of two groups, either Naha-te or Shuri-te, with various sub styles branching from these. Often, though not exclusively, *Sanchin* is considered the 'root' form taught within Naha based styles such as Uechi and Goju-ryu, whereas *Naihanchi* is the kata of more Shuri influenced styles. Both forms however have been known on Okinawa since ancient times, possibly even before the arrival of Kwan Ku in 1756 who is widely recognised as starting the Tode hybrid that would become karate.

Today the two forms are mostly taught in separate systems but it seems likely that if you go back far enough both *Naihanchi* and *Sanchin* would have been taught together because whereas the former develops an ideal physique upon which to develop boxing skills the latter develops the *hara* and breathing method to support them. In short, *Naihanchi* is the frame for Okinawan Karate and *Sanchin* the engine.

Where differences exist between versions of the same kata is like an echo of a seemingly now abandoned practice in which advanced students were actively encouraged by their teachers to alter the forms and make them their own. Thus no one version is right or wrong, they are simply different interpretations along a common theme.

During the afternoons, on days when I stayed close to BASE I would practise kata on the beach or in the sea. A habit I still enjoy today.

In some ways it stirs memories of those times I'd trained in the mountains, close to nature and with no one around; something I hadn't done in years. But on the beach, in the sea, your kata takes on a different aspect. You become aware of the rhythms of the tide and the pulse of the planet and on another level you have to work hard to maintain posture and proper breathing in tune with this rhythm.

Uehara Seikichi of the Motobu Udundi Te style used to practise in the sea. In an interview during his late nineties he recalled how he used to get into the water up to his neck and keep his posture still.

'I looked towards the horizon and used to sing and shout. I sometimes used to swallow the salt water, and the cold attacked my body. But I used to train like that three times a week. It was dangerous to do it every day since it could damage the respiratory system.'

One sunny afternoon Marcos and I were training on the beach. He'd returned from a week further up the island and his sensei had awarded him a nice hardwood *bo* staff as a leaving gift. We were doing what *bujin* had done on Naminoue for years; exchanging ideas, sharing and developing our training in a brotherhood spirit. At one point two Danish students from the hostel came down too. They were studying Goju-ryu and began with rehearsing kata while I showed Marcos some simple techniques from the Yamane-ryu *bojutsu* style Higa was teaching me.

Yamane-ryu is another 'family' tradition on Okinawa. It specialises in the use of the *rokushaku-bo* or 'six foot' staff. Unique in its approach the Yamane style uses a technique of sliding the weapon into lighting fast strikes reminiscent of the movements of a Pool cue. It's this technique that gives the style a deceptive way of manipulating the distance between an opponent and enables the skilled wielder to use the end of the weapon to strike pressure points and neutralise attacks. It evolves from spear fighting, most likely from Southern China.

What was interesting from that afternoon on the beach was that while Marcos and I began working unarmed defences against *bo* attacks, the Danish guys started sparring, and a dog, belonging to some locals, started snarling and barking. Not at us but the Danes.

It seemed that whereas Marcos and I were swinging a big stick and leading each other into Te-like rolls the others were clashing in true Goju form and, to the dog at least, it must have seemed the more aggressive of the two. I mean on a primitive, sense-orientated level.

The Danes had to stop after a short while through fear of being bitten. Yet all the while Marcos and I continued exchanging attacks un-affected. I reasoned it must have been an 'adrenaline' based thing. In their keen nature to train hard a sort of rivalry was flaring up between the Danes with each trying to 'score' points on the other. With spectators watching maybe ego's were getting bruised and they were getting beside themselves. In either case the dog was getting agitated.

As with the primitive aspects of body posturing and eye contact I'd witnessed with Mark in that carpark, and untold street fights in London bars, the adrenalised energy of the situation was palpable. At least to the fine tuned senses of a dog it was. To onlookers there probably wasn't much difference in what the four of us were doing, but our intentions were certainly different. Marcos and I were sharing and learning through give and take. The Danes had crossed the threshold of that and were being led to bettering one another in competition.

Martial arts training exercises like *Sanchin*, regardless of style or versions, are designed to increase sensitivity. Initially on a tactile basis for physical combat but also on more subtle levels like thoughts, intent, or even the pheromones given off in adrenalised situations. It's the reason why masters of old like Kishimoto Soko could detect when an unseen attacker was lurking in the shadows, waiting to pounce, or why the group I first travelled to Japan with spoke of detecting gamma-rays photons, even supernova exploding in deep space. *Ki*. Intent. Energy.

Essentially we are all receptors of Universe, made from the fabric of Universe. Understanding this point, knowing it, feeling it and experiencing it, is what empowers us to rise above the fear motivated behaviours of 'sitting with our backs to walls' and 'giving corners wide berths'. You come to realise that you don't have to live in anticipation of being attacked because when the time comes you'll feel the ripples of destructive thoughts around you before they even transmute into their physical equivalent. The purpose of your martial arts training then should be to hone these antennae-like receptors beyond merely feeling through tactile touch, or even beyond the hairs rising on the back of your neck. There are more than five senses; some are just incredibly subtle.

Besides. Fighting for the sake of fighting is a mugs game.

Matsuyama Park, about fifteen minutes walk from Naminoue, is the place where those who wanted to brag about their karate skill nearly two hundred years ago would go for challenge matches. The roads of Tsuji behind Naminioue, filled now as they were then with late night bars and prostitution, were also the stage of frequent fights and social unrest. Unlike today.

For the most part such '*kumite*' matches provided a means of developing the various styles and keeping the art alive, but after a time it became a nuisance and threatened social unrest. Deaths were not uncommon and authorities were called. Sometimes that made things worst. Like in the case of a low ranking official named Tokumine who bettered, or battered, thirty constables in a street brawl. Tokumine was eventually shipped off to the Yaeyama Islands far to the south as an 'undesirable'. Perhaps in the late 1800's Okinawa itself was becoming something of a place for undesirables to end up at for it was then on the periphery of the Japanese Empire, economically poor and considered something of a backwater country by those on the mainland.

In Matsuyama Park things got so bad that eventually a magistrate from Shuri-jo arrived one day to 'lay down the law'. Any who felt they could better him were welcome to try. When one such 'tough' stepped up to the mark the official drew his sword. "What's this?" The tough protested.

"Well you all like to fight, and fighting is a serious business. People lose their lives fighting so you should always be sure to fight for something worthwhile. I am fighting with a sword - are you ready to die?"

After that, the troubles in Matsuyama quietened down somewhat.

It's another martial art tale handed down by word of mouth but the Official from Shuri had a valid point. How many times do young men fly off the handle and cause trouble so easily, running in packs like feral dogs? The problems of such anti social behaviour are rife in many cities and towns around the world and much of the time someone uses a bottle as a weapon, pulls a knife or fires a gun. For what? Pride? Ego? Some misplaced sense of self-respect? Boredom?

A famous Okinawan poem says "Life is a treasure". Take the effort to guard it well.

*

After training late one night I was riding back through Asato and suddenly swerved dangerously through several lanes of traffic beneath Furujima station. The reason for my reckless road-sense wasn't an act of social disobedience but to shepherd a stray dog, dangerously running scared, away from the main flow of traffic and into the quieter side roads.

He had a loose length of frayed wire for a lead and a haphazard collar of leather and duct tape. You'd be forgiven for mistaking him as a homeless person's companion, except the homeless in Japan rarely keep animals. Okianwa has a problem with strays, and the parks at night are mewing with cats, but there was something about this fella that seemed out of place. Despite his shabby coat he was in reasonable health. He probably lived outside in a concrete yard and had managed to get himself free. I led him to a store and bought some hotdogs and water for him while I contemplated what to do.

Not far from the store was a shrine, and I had half a mind to leave him tied up there but for his affectionate and good mannered behaviour which seemed to demand something more. I had potentially just saved his life so why would I now put that aside and leave his survival to chance again?

Needing time to think I held his lead and continued cycling back towards the hostel. He kept perfect pace, never dashed off or pulled away. We stopped by the Eager Beaver bar and he waited beneath the sandwich-board sign as I went inside. Being a mostly expats bar several of the staff and customers were keen to help but no-one really knew how or what to do, so after a drink I rode with him back to the hostel.

The owners there already had a dog so I knew I couldn't take him in. Instead I went to a small garden and tied him to a bench while I went for some help from the staff. Again, being mostly young workers down from the mainland and perhaps knowing what it's like to have the support of other's around, they were genuinely concerned about the dogs welfare. We tried the police station but they only suggested taking him back where I found him and letting him find his way home.

Shoo, the manager of the hostel, spoke with the family that owned the business. They were happy to let the dog live under the eaves so long as it could get along with their existing dog. That wasn't likely. Their dog was old, a little grumpy and the doorway to the hostel was his territory.

There was a guest at the hostel, a formidable character called The Captain. Dressed in biker leathers with an 'easy rider' parked outside and a long *tenugui* tied about his head he was fiercely patriotic and spoke no English. But he also had an instant attachment to the dog. I was told he'd once owned one similar who would sit on the gas tank of his motorbike while he toured Japan years before. Now he owned a shop in Osaka where he painted leathers like a tattoo artist and he contemplated taking the dog on.

By 2am, a small group of us were leading the two dogs to the beach.

"Let them fight. It might seem cruel but they must fight, to learn their place." The plan was that the dogs would have a hurried scuffle and one would assert it's dominance over the other. Then, hopefully, they could live together at the hostel. Reluctantly I agreed but it was ultimately a flawed plan. The older dog was already the dominant one, the other was nervous and backing away, it had no fight in it, what was the point? Besides, as both dogs aged they would forever be challenging and reasserting dominance periodically.

After a minute of snarling, snapping, salivating jaws, met with a confused defence and fearful whining, I thrust a leg between the two and pulled them apart by the scruff. This wasn't the solution.

Walking my new friend further up the beach The Captain tried to intervene. We couldn't understand each other so someone translated.

"He says he will sleep with him tonight on the beach." I shook my head no. "I will stay with him tonight." The concept stunned them a little.

"Why would you do that? It will get cold out here tonight, it might not be safe." I smiled at the ridiculousness of that argument and nodded to The Captain.

"Tell him, I've been thinking. When I saved the dog from the road this evening it was a choice. I chose to save his life. Not just in that moment but for the future too. I'm responsible for him, so I will stay out here tonight, and tomorrow I will find a more longterm solution."

Measuring me with wide eyes, the frown of confusion on The Captain's face softened as our friend translated what I'd said. It was uncomfortable for both of them to let me, a visitor, sleep rough in their country. The police would always ignore a Japanese but a foreigner would more likely get picked up. But I wasn't arguing about it and it wasn't exactly my first experience of sleeping rough in Japan either. After a last attempt to persuade me otherwise The Captain smiled, bowed, and gave me a firm half-hug, a rare act of affection from a strong Japanese male. Particularly one who doesn't speak a word of English. But then sometimes words are overrated. The eyes and body language speak volumes.

Finding a quiet spot tucked away from any prying eyes I sat with the dog curled by my side and eventually laid down and drifted into a light sleep thinking of home.

> *On a journey,*
> *resting on the beach with blades of grass as my pillow,*
> *even in sleep never can I forget being beside my sweetheart.*
> *The beach plovers cry "chuichuina."*
> HAMACHIDORI

The following day I signed the dog over to a Pound who could only safeguard him for five days before they'd destroy him. I posted flyers asking for a home and had everyone I could spread the word to anyone they knew. The more people involved improved his chance of living. My fallback plan was that if nothing came up I would collect him before the five days were up and take him out to the farms outside of Naha looking for a home.

As fate would have it a small rehoming centre not far from the Bugeikan had picked up the story, paid his release fees and re-homed him with an employee in Okinawa City. Unlike many dogs in Okinawa, he would sleep inside a house from now on. A dog named Shen.

18
FM21
"Once we meet and talk,
we are brothers and sisters"

Higa sensei was drunk. With an infectious laugh he reversed the grip I held upon his lapel, swayed out of the way of my punch to his face, and leaned next to me with an arm about my side as if we were the best of old friends. You couldn't see it but my wrist was now trapped in a painful lock in the small of my back which made me teeter on my toes with a grimacing face.

Rolling his head he hiccuped and kept by my side, leading me left and right with the manipulation of the technique. "Sorry mister Porrice Officer" he began to explain, "my furiendu is drunk! It's okay, I take him home!"

Higa sensei was drunk, but he hadn't touched a drop of alcohol.

"Side by side, Joel-san. Not 'face to face', 'Side by side!' Hai?" Between twinges of pain, shooting through my nervous system like electric, I nodded whilst spasmodically tapping the side of my leg in submission.

'Side by side' was the lesson of the day. It could be found in the technique he just pulled on me, but more than that it meant 'don't fight'. That in *bujutsu* we must try to make friends out of enemies because most fights start over the most ridiculous of reasons anyway. And besides, it's better to keep your enemies closer than friends.

Also, in crowded locations, fighting can become infectious, like laughter, so when someone tries to hit you, you should simply avoid their blow and deescalate the situation by applying this 'side by side' approach. Appearing as 'friends with a misunderstanding' we can lead the aggressor away with hidden *tuiti* techniques.

This is what Te is like. Neutralising aggression and preserving life, not destroying it. I remember being on a course one weekend in England for an Okinawan style of karate. The group was friendly and trained hard yet the visiting teacher from abroad would insist on demonstrating techniques with bellicose language that included: "If I wanted to, I could kill them now, break their neck, snap an arm or crush their skull. But I'm a nice guy, I don't want to do that, so maybe I'd just pop an eye out or kick their kneecaps away." None of which sounded like he was seeking to nurture a friendship but all of which was likely to seed a blood feud for violent reprisals.

Uehara used to say, "When you enter a fight you potentially dig two graves, yours and your opponent's." What it meant was, even if you win the fight and take your opponent's life, his relatives or someone is going to come after you. Karma.

Anko Itosu, the Okinawan master who brought karate into the school system once wrote:

> *'Never attack a lone adversary. If one meets a villain or a ruffian one should not use karate but simply parry and step aside.'*

Before it became his dojo Uehara Seikichi used to run a bar that catered for American GI's. Sometimes, when soldiers refused to leave, Mrs Uehara would call upstairs for her husband's assistance. Obligingly he would come down, grin, smile and laugh with the nuisance soldiers and then offer to shake their hand. If you've ever been lucky enough to feel, or even 'see', Uehara's *tuiti* in action then you will understand what I mean when I say 'it was time to go'.

Releasing my hand, Higa walked away and I rubbed my sore wrist. This lesson had started half an hour earlier with a series of Seido stretches that blended breath and movement into one fluid workout to release stress and tension from the mind and body. A fluid mind needs a supple body.

Higa's level of flexibility is on a par with some of the more advanced of yoga exponents and his appearance is easily twenty, maybe thirty, years younger than his real age of nearly eighty. In fact, youthfulness had long been the third marker by which I had come to seek teacher's worth training under. The reason for this is that if a martial artists focusses too heavily on hard, adrenalised workouts then it taxes the body and damages the soft tissues of the joints. Furthermore, an excess of adrenalin in the system not only damages the immune system, it also hardens the muscles, tightens the ligaments and prematurely ages skin. There are a lot of karate sensei in the world who actually look older than they are, so my advice is find the ones that look younger. They have something worth learning. I don't mean this in a vain sense, but rather because their techniques will be of a higher level and more likely to release endorphins over adrenalin.

After the Seido routine Higa put on some music and we went into free-form, or 'natural movement'. Armed with folding red fans we began swaying and, in a sense, dancing to the music with an intoxicated vibe. The whole thing became like a soft form of tai-chi, albeit more fluid and slightly quicker in pace, and the movements, though appearing to an onlooker as dance, were actually effective self-defence sequences teaching throws, sweeps, strikes and kicks.

The song was an old 'Okinawan blues' track, which seemed to be amongst one of Higa's favourites. The movements were not choreographed though, he was 'channelling'. I know this because we always started these type of lessons from a meditative state with no intention of moving in a particular way. Actually, before the song had started Higa stood ahead of me and went into a similar trance as he does at the beginning of his spiritual ceremonies. The 'energy' then moves through him, and the techniques are spontaneous. These are *kamiwaza*; divine techniques.

I didn't need to guess which *kami* was in attendance because I sensed it before we started. It was Bugei-no-kami, the '*kami*' of martial arts that sometimes appears in dragon form and sometimes as the Old Sage who's name was once Motobu Seijin.

It wasn't really Higa who was drunk, it was the *kami*. It's a strange sensation too, because without choreography I realised I wasn't actually 'following' his lead but rather moving with him. Much like those dreams I'd had years earlier which had brought me here.

Our movements swayed, stumbled and tripped, all in unison and with a sort of jovial drunkenness. Sometimes we'd spin about and drive a kick upwards beneath the fan, or spiral downwards snapping it shut with a loud 'crack!' We'd trip and fall into a forward roll, sometimes springing back to our feet with a punch or at other times rolling into leg sweeps and then leaping into the air. Before the end we found ourselves exactly back upon the spots we started from despite having moved about the entire floor.

Takimiyagi had once said that the 'drunken style' is the second highest method of Udundi technique, it's approach makes for an unpredictable defence with a softness of movement that can shift instantly into a pin-point strike. Beyond drunken-style, in Udundi, is the mystical 'Dance Hand of the Lords' but with Higa it is simply free-form, or 'natural' movement.

I am aware that others approaching Higa for tuition are often turned away at the door or directed to one of his sons who has a dojo in Itoman. Mostly this is because he has retired from teaching or because others request only to learn a specific aspect form one of the eight martial styles he holds a master grade in.

After training one night, another long-term student of Higa's took me for a meal at a restaurant.

"Higa sensei isn't really a closed teacher but he is hidden. There are very few he will teach these days. Most come with an agenda and want only to learn a certain 'thing' or style. They only want to learn what a 'specific' teacher taught him, or his father. Sometimes these are entertained and given a little to go away with, but never the full picture. Higa sensei is a little 'old school' in this regard and holds back a lot."

She was one of the privileged few to train with Higa these days. There were only four of us in total. Her husband teaches Motobu Udundi but because it is difficult to train under a loved one she is honoured to be taught by Higa.

"For you he is very open. He has said that he is very pleased you have come and that he intends to teach you everything he can." She smiled as I awkwardly received the compliment. "This is because he has seen in your heart. You came very open and honest."

Usually Higa's English is limited and my Japanese too basic, so much of our 'transmission of knowledge' is what is termed 'heart to heart'.

One day Higa was teaching an intricate point about a strategy of a technique. He explained in Japanese whilst demonstrating on me, and his daughter smiled curiously from the sofa from where she was watching. "Do you understand what he is saying?"

"No. Not really. But I can 'feel' what he means." Thinking I meant physically she re-framed her question. "Yes but to understand the technique, like it's timing, rhythm or correct application is different than just feeling it.

"I know. I can't fully explain it but when your father teaches me I 'feel' it in my heart and see pictures in my mind. It's more like telepathy or 'emotional-knowing'."

Spoken language, whether it be English or Japanese is perhaps insufficient to describe this phenomena.

*

FM21. Wednesday. 13:30. A week earlier Higa had asked me to meet him in Urazoe at the offices of a mainstream radio station. He wanted me to appear on a popular show with him to discus training in martial arts on Okinawa. Over the course of an hour the format of the show took the form of an interview with the DJ fielding questions about my training and discussing key points with Higa about traditional natural exercises like karate, kobudo and Seido for health.

After a brief introduction I was asked about my background in martial arts, how I'd first learnt the basics of judo from my father and then studied Shotokan, Tai chi, yoga and Okinawan *bujutsu*. I talked about working as a shiatsu practitioner in the UK and how, for me, the martial arts had become more than just a means of combat but a life art that brought union to the heart, mind and spirit. We discussed Higa's approach to *bujutsu* and the importance of building harmonious relationships with others to promote peace without conflict. A non confrontational martial art summed up well by an old Okinawan proverb that says: *'Once we meet and talk, we are brothers and sisters.'*

Higa was asked about his own martial arts upbringing, his study of Yamane-ryu *bojutsu*, the essence of Seido and advice on developing *ki* for maintaining health.

Towards the end of the show, much to my surprise, he announced in near perfect English how pleased he was with my progress. How my quality of movement and honest approach was of a level he'd not seen in anyone for a great many years and that, for this reason, it was his intention to teach me everything he could.

Bowing my head I thanked him and reiterated my desire to remain his student. In a few more weeks I'd be returning to England, but this would be the first trip of many.

Just a few evenings before, I was meditating in the dojo and had a sense of feeling I'd not felt before. That now, having found Higa, there was no other teacher I wanted to learn from. That it had become my intention to train with him until the end.

The training I'd received so far was a lot but it was just the surface, I knew that.

Having studied a lineage chart of the styles preserved at the Bugeikan I came to realise that in 2001 Higa sensei was awarded the *menkyo kaiden*, 'Successor Certificate', of Hanashiro Chomo's Shorin Ryu karate lineage. This was worth knowing more about. Whereas Funakoshi travelled to the mainland to further karate in the early 1920s, his *sempai*, Hanashiro remained on Okinawa teaching the kata their teacher Itosu had taught them, unaltered. All of the original forms taught by Funakoshi that formed the basis of Shotokan are preserved by Higa sensei at the Bugeikan in their purest versions. Higa learnt them via a personal teacher of his named Kanzou Nakadankari.

After the show I travelled back to Shuri alone. I wanted to wander through the Palace grounds once more and revel in the splendour of its reconstructed architecture. Having been ravaged by war Shurijo had been built anew. Yes it was a tourist attraction now but more than that it's new lease of life was overseeing an era of peace once again.

Practising a few kata in the quiet sanctuary of the Benzaiten temple, a shrine for the goddess of eloquence, music and art. I sat and contemplated my journey so far. I thought back to those first days arriving in Tokyo, the fanatical lot and The Grandmaster who controlled time. There was the kind generosity Mr Sawada had afforded me, and my friend Masakazu, who I'd long since lost contact with but knew had become a successful doctor somewhere in Tokyo. I smiled thinking about the Old Man in the park and that first hint he gave me that that mystical art Funakoshi once wrote about, 'Okinawa-te', had somehow survived into the twentieth century. The words of Funakoshi's poem echoed in my thoughts once more; *'to search for the old is to understand the new'*. His teacher, Asato, had probably once stood exactly where I was right now, enjoying the solitude of the small temple in the middle of a pond.

I'd come a long way for sure but I couldn't rightly say what I'd found. What was Te really? To me it seemed a distinct artform from the karate I'd learnt. The very mechanics and dynamics of it differed greatly from the karate in Kanazawa's dojo, even from the styles of karate here on the island too. But there were similarities as well; snippets of movements and combative strategies that stood out from the rest. The techniques of punching and kicking in Motobu Udundi and at the Bugeikan were considered too light by the majority of karate exponents I had exchanged with. They certainly were unlike any techniques they'd encountered before. And yet the dynamics of those movements shared closer links with the 'sporting' styled karate of today. Moving on the toes, constantly shifting weight, attacking with the lead, no blocks, and so on.

One thing I found interesting was that none of the teachers of Motobu ryu, or Higa at the Bugeikan, seemed to ever use the term 'Te' to describe their art. Even senior karate teachers on the island will tell you Te doesn't exist, but it does really. Sort of. Was this another case of Okinawan cultural amnesia?

When I asked Higa sensei what Te was, he answered somewhat philosophically, "Te is karate, karate is Te." Refining my enquiry I asked "what then is Motobu Udundi?" At this he simply smiled and waved his hands around in the *kashashi* movement of dance. "Motobu Udundi is this." He wasn't being derogatory. In his youth Higa had trained under Uehara Seikichi for many years and was awarded a *hanshi* grade by him. In a way I felt he was telling me 'Motobu Udundi' is just 'a part' of what you're learning, and it isn't everything. In a zen-like way he was cutting through all the nonsense and giving me a direct answer by revealing that the core of Udundi strategy is found within the changing hand movements of Okinawan dance. Three simple waves of the hand.

Takamiyagi said that the term 'Te' is a suffix used to describe a certain technique or method. As in *kashin-te*, *ogami-te* or *tuiti*. Other writers, with no grounding in either Motobu-ryu or at the Bugeikan, have suggested that Te was simply a rudimentary form of boxing on the island that favoured the closed fist. But that doesn't really hold because the closed fist of Te comes from gripping a weapon, be it a sword, spear or bow, and uses the thumb as the primary striking surface not the knuckles. Besides, most unarmed techniques in Te use the open hand.

It has also been suggested that a similar antiquated term was '*Tigwa*' but *ti'gwa* is simply an informal, and slightly derisive way, of saying 'Te' in the generic sense of 'martial arts'. A mother might say to her son going out to train "are you off to play *ti'gwa?*"

Perhaps one of the loudest voices proclaiming 'Te' to be a distinct martial art is Mark Bishop. In many ways his first book *Okinawan Karate* brought a far greater awareness of Te into the twentieth century than any other person or group I know of.

What made me so certain it exists? I feel Te is a distinct martial art because everyone who comes to try it from an advanced background in karate, regardless of style, finds themselves like a fish out of water for the first couple of sessions. Yes there are some similarities, but the differences are greater. Footwork in Te is liberated, light and springy. There are few fixed-fighting drills because the training is free-form in nature. The way of striking is different. Kicks and strikes come from the lead hand rather than the reverse. There is no *hikite* or 'pulling' technique. There are no blocks, no stances and no kata. Anything resembling a 'karate kata' in Te is no older than two hundred years, and in Motobu Udundi they were added as 'auxiliary' training aids to help migrating karate-ka adapt to Te training methods. The movements of karate kata are methodical and formed from linear thought-patterns whereas the movements of Te are liberated and spontaneous.

Te is an enigma, but it does exist. In order to describe the art in the eyes of Okinawans I found the term Ryukyu Bujutsu more appropriate. This, in some way, helped to define the art as being different to karate or kobudo. In conversations with friends at the hostel or about town the term Ryukyu Bujutsu conjured the right images in mind. None however realised that such an art could still be learnt in today's age. If Te were more widely known then perhaps there would be a resurgence of it on its native homeland where today it remains so little known.

Crossing back over the small wooden bridge I left the temple behind and made my way down into town. Despite everything I had discovered so far there was still one more thing I wanted to explore before flying out in a couple of weeks time. Where, if it existed as I was saying it did, did this 'Te' come from? What was it's origin?

19
Change
"Change comes from within."

One balmy evening I went to meet a contact at the Eager Beaver bar in Makishi. When I arrived I don't think either of us was quite what the other expected. He was older than I thought, and I was younger.

Hideki had been introduced to me via email before leaving England. Having expressed an interest in Ryukyuan history he wanted to meet to discus my 'theory' of Te being a unique martial art of Okinawa. When I arrived the barmaid nodded to an older gentleman sitting in the corner with a glass of wine.

Wearing a pressed shirt and bowtie, a pair of trousers and braces, Hideki cut an eccentric demeanour that at once made him both interesting and enjoyable to be around. Perhaps in his sixties, he had a rounded paunch and shifted from one contemplative pose to another as we chatted about such diverse topics as *Wako* pirates, castles, Okinawan theatre, dance and martial arts.

Early in the meeting he slid a pale blue paper envelope across the table with 'UNIVERSITY OF THE RYUKYUS FACULTY OF EDUCATION' printed upon its front. "This is for you to open after we have met" he added, with the hint of an enigmatic smile playing upon his lips. Hideki spoke perfect English but in a sort of melodic singing like way that made me feel he was a from a former time. He asked about my training and the places I'd visited on the island whilst investigating my 'theory', and of course, 'did I still feel that Te was an Okinawan martial art?'

Cupping his chin and nodding with humming filler sounds of interest he let me explain where I was at. Then, taking out a slender folded fan he snapped it open with a flick of the wrist and wafted the air upon his face.

"Yes, yes. Fascinating. Truly fascinating. But can a martial art like this really come from such a small island, like Okinawa? Don't you think that it must have come from somewhere else? China perhaps?"

Actually I didn't. I put forward that karate had significantly been influenced by Chinese kung-fu but that Te was clearly of a far older period. To this Hideki totally agreed but he pressed a little further.

"Okinawa is so small. I think, to develop the type of martial art you are describing, it would need to have come from a country that had centuries of experience in warfare. These things do not just simply 'appear.'"

I could agree with that. But despite Okinawa's small size it has an extensive collection of castle structures and had, for hundreds of years, been divided by three principal states that fought relentlessly with each other over the limited natural resources and deep water bays around the island.

These *gusuku* castles were not mere forts. They boasted magnificent ramparts constructed of limestone and coral and they utilised the geographical strengths of their surroundings by hugging the contours of cliffs and hills. The *gusuku* of Okinawa demonstrate a remarkably advanced understanding of military science and they differed significantly from those found in Korea, China and Japan; although borrowed from them too.

When the ancient Japanese state of Yamato began extending its sphere of influence south of Kyushu, around AD700, it succeeded in pacifying the islands to the north and west of

Okinawa, yet curiously Okinawa does not appear in ancient records until a good fifty years later, despite it being the largest and most resource rich island in the region. Had the Yamato raiding expeditions found it to already be well defended by a war-like people putting up organised defence?

The earliest mention of the Ryukyu's in Chinese records describes an expeditionary force meeting fierce resistance from locals as they hastily retreated back to their ships with heavy losses.

I had to agree with Hideki though. We simply don't know for sure. Unlike Hideki however I did not feel the major influence on Te was from China. My research was leading more to ancient Japan and some of the earliest forms of *bujutsu* to emerge there.

After a couple of drinks our meeting wound down to an agreeable end. That is, in the spirit of positive academic research, we agreed to disagree. As a parting shot Hideki laid down a gauntlet; a challenge of sorts.

"Kikaijima. Look into the island of Kikaijima, 'that' is a very interesting place." He smiled.

Before he left, Hideki introduced me to another patron of the bar. Nice Guy Paul.

Nice Guy Paul was interested to hear about an 'older history' of Okinawa because during his nearly ten years on the island teaching English he had only really heard about WWII. Paul would make trips around the island on his bicycle to explore old pill-boxes, re-work campaign maps from the library and read about the American Invasion of 1945, 'The Battle for Okinawa' At the time he just hadn't heard much about Ryukyuan history. Sadly a lot of the younger Okinawan generation are the same which is a shame because for me Okinawa's history is in many ways a microcosm of world history, and the story of human evolution itself.

Having come through the monstrous destruction of WWII the island has re-invented itself with valuable lessons the rest of the world could learn. Lessons about how a nation can exist at peace without spending ridiculous amounts of money on bettering ways of killing greater numbers of people.

The truth is that as we move into this twenty-first century the world will progressively become a borderless place. During this time it will be important to preserve unique expressions of culture in order to maintain identity, but it is only by recognising that 'different' does not automatically equate to 'better' that we can really start accepting one another as neighbours. Cultural expression begins with sharing and mutual respect, not by assuming cultural superiority.

As this world becomes more unified, resources can be pooled and used more efficiently; which has really been the cause of all major wars anyway. Governments in the future will need to let go of past thought patterns and power structures. Like karate kata, they are good to get so far but should ultimately be discarded for the tools they are when the time is right. In order for the human race to move forward, as a family, nations must start looking at ways of improving the quality of life of their citizens without exploiting others for financial gain in the process.

Okinawa has already embraced this concept. Given greater autonomy from Japan proper it could exercise it even more. Other countries around the world are also changing their ways, focusing their wealth on 'livingry' over weaponry. A changing tide is coming.

Nice Guy Paul seemed genuinely interested to hear about the Shō Dynasty, the Sanzan period of civil war and the *gusuku* sites of Okinawa. I imagine he started to see the parts of the island he'd passed in ruin with fresh eyes that brought them to life with images of *bushi* knights on horseback, archers lining the parapets and bloody battle's of a different kind on the flatlands and riverbanks around the island.

Through Nice Guy Paul I was able to meet Mrs Itokazu, a Professor of History at the University of Ryukyu, who generously gave me her time during my final week on the island to research the origins of the *noro* priestess class which I felt held the clue to the origin of Te.

When I got back to the hostel that night I opened the envelope from Hideki and laughed. Inside were several pamphlets and documents of his role with the Okinawa Cultural Association which presents annual displays of Ryukyu Dance, Music and Karate around the world. He had utterly defeated me that evening and I burned with embarrassment because Hideki Takeda had failed to mention he was a senior 8th dan of Goju-ryu known for his unique displays of karate in which he defends from attacks whilst sitting in the relaxed cross-legged posture of Okinawan custom. A true *bujin* master who expressed the finer qualities of the martial code.

*

My final session at the Bugeikan came one Friday afternoon. I cycled up the hill to the Gibo crossroads and arrived early.

My intention was to enjoy a good hour and half stretching out and meditating before Isyado turned up to mercilessly drill me in his fashion. I guess great minds really do think a like though, because Isyado was already there. With a smile I got changed and went straight to it. *Naihanchi, Sanchin, Nidan bu*, punches, kicks, throws, more throws, more. More.

Standing before me now, with a bokken covered with pipe-insulating foam, Isyado's eyes watched my every movement. The goal of the exercise was to 'avoid and enter'. That is, avoid being hit by the sword and simultaneously enter into his space to strike him.

Attempt after attempt I failed, receiving hits to my arms, collarbones or back as Isyado caught me with every pass. Mrs Higa, her daughters and grand-daughter watched from the sofa at the back with grimacing faces and flinches with each failure. More faces started to turn up, my fellow training partners and Higa's sons Kiyotomo and Kiyohiro. Feeling the exhaustion of an hour's intensive training in basics beforehand, I sighed and shook off the fatigue. Relax. Relax. Relax. The evening air was close and muggy.

Entering a calmer state of mind I wiped the slate clean on my previous attempts and now stared through Isyado. I was light on my feet, feeling his breathing and mirroring the sway of his own movements. Sensing his attack I burst forward and contorted into a fast strike towards his chest avoiding the predicted upward cut of the sword. Turning on the spot I continued through to strike again as the sword now came diagonally down on the return. Again I twisted and sculpted my body to avoid the movement. Not a conscious response, a natural one.

Ducking and rolling away from his third cut it narrowly missed my back and so pushing into the balls of my feet I rushed back on the return and leapt effortlessly within the arcing movement of the weapon with an open hand reaching to the *tenugui* tied about his forehead.

That rag of a towel was something of a trademark for my *sempai* and our audience gasped in shock. Had I wanted to I could have snatched that towel clean from his head. It was the closest I'd ever got but I didn't need to take it. He knew it too.

Turning to face each other squarely, my face burning and drenched in sweat, he lowered the sword and smiled with a broad grin. I'd won. It wasn't so much that I had avoided being hit or even that I had succeeded in entering his space that made me happy though. It was his grin. A month earlier I had told Mrs Higa that I intended to make Isyado smile. His stern and serious face had been something of a talking point in conversation, and they said it wasn't possible. His genuine grin and mild shock was my sweet victory.

But if I thought that was the end of my training that evening I was mistaken. A few minutes later Higa sensei came up and nodded as he sat upon his seat, positioned as it was like something of a throne at the front of the shrine area.

Turning up early had been a big mistake because now, at our 'usual' time Higa wanted to see a run through of everything we had covered to date. Isyado had a look that said he wanted to explain he'd already done this. But of course, he didn't. He did look a little guilty though as he stepped to the side and called out the instructions. ... *Naihanchi, Sanchin, Nidan bu*, punches, kicks, throws, more throws, more. More.

Then came kobudo *kata, nunchaku, bo, yari, naginata, katana*; flail, staff, spear, glaive, sword. All the while more faces kept arriving, members of the congregation, faces of trainees I'd not met but had seen before in old videos of the Bugeikan, even the local priest. I was shattered and close to dropping from exhaustion. This kind of training, in the humid Naha heat, was more like when I trained with Sawada sensei in Tokyo. The problem was I was eighteen then. I was in my thirties now.

Masato showed up, my training partner. We'd only trained together a few times a week but he had been a good support in my early days, offering me lifts home in his car after particularly gruelling sessions. Together we now practised *jissen kumite*, exchanging both empty handed and weapon attacks. Then a round with Isyado.

Eventually things started to ease down. Higa sensei came and taught two different methods of entering an attack and redirecting the opponent into a throw before moving on to Seido, the breathing and movement based exercise that opens the body and leads to free-form or 'natural' movement. For this everyone present joined in.

I had come to learn that, where Motobu Udundi technique had been preserved in semi-secrecy within the refined Court Styled dances of *kumiodori*, the Te taught by the Higa family had a far older connection that linked directly back to the *noro*, priestesses of the Royal Court. The *noro* utilised the same three hand gestures of Te as part of their ritualised prayer ceremony. The role of such women reached far back into the earliest periods of Okinawan culture. Prayer-hand, twist-hand and push-hand. These three gestures are the means through which intent is brought into its physical reality, and in combat, through combination, they can lead to limitless defences.

Kumiodori became the vehicle through which Te technique was codified and carried through the eighteenth to twentieth centuries by members of the great warrior clans of Shuri. But at the highest level of Motobu Udundi is a now lost practice known as *Anjikata-no-Me-kata* or 'Dance Hand of the Lords'. An old poem by Choyo reads:

> *"Never think of just observing, Anjikata-no-Me-kata, for technique compounds technique and the more the secrets come to light."*

What this meant is that the real techniques of Te are not so much to be found in the 'outer' form but more in the 'internal' dance of the body.

It gets deeper than that though. The very movements of this form provided a means through which members of the Motobu clan could unravel and overcome ancestral notices, or curses, upon their bloodline; karmically speaking.

To fully understand this concept is to delve deeper into the religion of Ancestors Worship and Okinawan concepts relating to the transcendence of psychosomatic illnesses and addictions passed down successive generations. Karma is social and genetic. You are your father's father and the fathers of the future. In very simple terms the actions of your grandfather have played a significant role in your life whether you are aware of them or not. And not just through the course of reproduction. This is why genealogy played such an important role within Okinawan aristocratic society and also what keeps Ancestors Worship alive. Not too dissimilar perhaps to the ceremony of baptism in Christianity. Movement and intent becomes prayer.

People say Uehara Seikichi failed to learn *Anjikata-no-Me-kata* from his teacher Choyo Motobu, but in a sense, he didn't need to; it wasn't related to his karma. Uehara wasn't descended from the Royal bloodline like the Motobu's were. To be sure, *Anjikata-no-Me-kata* was a physical, mental and spiritual practice of cleaning the karmic channels of the Royal line, it possibly wasn't even a structured 'form' like those in karate might think either.

Higa's 'natural' or 'free-movement' coming from Seido is, in a sense, his expression of *Anjikata-no-Me-kata*, and shares remarkable similarities to the hidden *noro* ceremonies that took place in the sacred grove sites about the island. The senior *noro* office of *Kikoe Okimi* was a position held only by a close female relative to the reigning king, usually his sister. Interestingly, the former residence of the *Kikoe Okimi* is located just across the street from the former Bugeikan dojo; that same spot where I first had those vibrating sensations upon arriving on the island. When Higa's father first bought the plot he determined, through deep meditation, that a martial art like Te had once been taught on the same site by a nobleman named Motobu Seijin over a thousand years earlier. But who can say?

Gichin Funakoshi used to say that all one needed to do was practise the kata and that eventually, to the right student, the meaning of the movements would reveal themselves. In a way I suspect *Anjikata-no-Me-kata* is a bit like this.

As my final session at the Bugeikan came to a close, those gathered congregated into one of the largest meetings I'd seen in my time on the island. Higa sensei's mother, who presided over the nightly ceremonies from a chair to his right, smiled and commented on how red my face was, and how she was going to miss me arriving early each day and calling out to her as I entered the home.

I looked around at everyone who was in attendance. The place had a strange 'family-like' atmosphere. Yes there were those who'd come for what really could be described in western terms as something of a church. Yet within this 'church' there were also martial artists, only a handful, who trained diligently and hard. They were custodians of sorts, not only of the Higa Family style but the teachings of other famous *bujin* like Hanashiro Chomo, Yamane Pechin, Tachimura, Kishimoto, Uehara Seikichi and Chozo Nakama.

Before the ritualised opening ceremony began Higa reflected upon my time in the dojo and praised my efforts. With a warm smile he stood up and presented me with a certificate, hand brushed in fluid kanji, bordered with two golden phoenix's and stamped with a red seal. Above the characters for my name were two kanji that read Go-dan, the 5th degree level of black belt.

With a heavy feeling, knowing that I would be leaving the following day, I looked around and took in the congratulating wishes and faces of the group. There was real happiness here, real pride and support. I knew this was a closing chapter of sorts upon a long journey to discover the old in order to understand the new. Only now I was no longer sure what was old and what was new. Somewhere along the way a change had taken place, but I couldn't exactly be sure where or what that change really was.

The next day I'd be heading home to England. There would be other adventures in the future but for now it was time to return home and slowly digest all I'd learnt. It takes time to absorb the meanings of lessons from such great teachers as I'd met on Okinawa, time to absorb them fully into your being. Anko Itosu once wrote:

'Karate cannot be learnt quickly, like a slow moving bull, that eventually walks a thousand miles, if one studies seriously every day, in three or four years one will understand what karate is about. The very shape of one's bones will change.'

Where was my change?

Change comes from within. Naturally.

Epilogue
The Old, the new
'Without health nothing else matters'

In Okinawa, karate is very serious. Teachers, good ones that still have something worth learning, are hard to find and guard their techniques closely. They don't just teach anyone who pays and they won't be found on any pre-organised bus tour around the island. The relationship between teacher and student develops organically. Not manufactured or fake, but open and pure.

In the early stages the teacher is likely to setup a number of tests to see if a candidate is of good character. Judge whether they can be trusted or not? If they have a 'good heart'. Basically, to be sure they are genuine and have the determination to succeed.

When Seiken Shukumine petitioned Soko Kishimoto for instruction, the master pondered by the fireplace stoking the embers. Then, without warning, he turned and threw the hot poker straight at Seiken who adroitly dodged it. Kishimoto accepted him as a student.

The test here, and for stories like it, is that the one seeking apprenticeship didn't get angered, didn't fly into a rage or seek vengeance. He also demonstrated a natural alertness. The martial arts of old are full of such stories.

Other tests could include setting daily chores such as sweeping the yard, digging trenches or cutting wood. Or washing cars, painting fences and sanding decks. Just as in the 1980's film *The Karate Kid* the chores not only served as a means of concentrating thought and action into one, but held hidden purpose too, a deeper meaning, a root technique.

In Japan, a traditional apprenticeship with any sensei, whether it be in karate, sword making or bonsai is likely to last around five years. In Bonsai the first three years might be spent maintaining the gardens, sweeping paths and watering potted trees. The techniques of cultivating, clipping and training come later. In this way a natural hierarchy forms. Respect and trust are earned over time whereas all too often in todays fast-paced world it is given more freely and abused just as quickly.

In karate one such character test could be to go out drinking one evening. A stooge would be invited too. Someone you've probably never met before, a local perhaps, who freely plays the fool and can never say no to 'just one more drink'. The trap set, the sensei will let the night unfold and quietly observe. In most cases it wont be the teacher themselves but a senior or close contact who escorts you for the evening. They probably wont let you pay a penny so money wont be what governs your behaviour, it's all down to you. Will you know your limits? Or will you fail and follow the stooge into drunkenness?

Why does this happen? Simple. In the wrong hands karate can be very destructive. Deadly. If a student were to get into a fight and seriously injure or kill another person the ultimate blame would fall upon the teacher. Certainly it would be the student who is in trouble with the law, but socially and karmically it is the teacher who will 'lose face' and take on shame; their reputation marred and judge of character doubted.

The teacher leads, the student follows.

This is why 'secret' techniques existed, and still do. Most of the time a sensei will choose a 'successor' to their style, someone who will preserve and further the schools lineage in accordance with the founder's wishes. Secret techniques are revealed to successor students over the course of time. This student might not be the most senior graded in the dojo. Often they are not. Neither does being a son or daughter grant instant 'successorship', although many are.

For the rest of the students the techniques might be slightly altered. Inner meanings remain unspoken and the most advanced methods glossed over. This is why many people take the time to research the lineages of their chosen styles so closely and strive to find authentic sensei. As one karate-ka once told me: "In karate, lineage is key."

Of course very often one mans secret is another's common knowledge and the majority of secret techniques are really just subtle ones that aren't so easily observed by the naked eye. For example. If someone were to apply a choke or strangle hold and you wanted to give yourself another thirty to fifty seconds to escape you could tuck your chin down and push your tongue to the roof of your mouth. The tongue is a strong muscle and this action would enable you to keep your windpipe open. With training you can continue breathing through your nose. That is a secret technique.

Another one, passed to me years later, concerns the alignment of the wrist in what is typically described as an 'inside forearm block', *uchi-ude-uke*. Here the secret was again for the preservation of ones own health. The end shape of the technique, being similar to the upward position when performing a dumbbell lift, bends the wrist in such a way that it applies excessive pressure upon a pressure-point located at the junction where the thumb meets the wrist. Over years of practice this feeds back tension into the nerves of the neck and can have a detrimental effect on wellbeing. The secret then is to perform the technique with the middle knuckle of the index finger aligned with the radial bone of the forearm. A subtle difference of less than a centimetre. As you can see, sometimes secret techniques are really just 'hidden' techniques.

For the right student, there are no secret or hidden techniques.

*

As I think back over this journey, '*searching for the old to understand the new*', I am left with a question. What, if anything, remains of Te in karate today? From my vantage point it is clear to me that several techniques of Te exist within karate, but it is only when they are allowed to be explored freely that they will truly benefit the individual. Kept within the confines of a basic form they will not reveal their true intent and trying to apply them without understanding will be like pushing a round peg into a square hole, or hammering nails with a spanner. You'll get some effect but it won't be the best result.

When seeking to unravel the Te hidden or preserved within karate, aside from the principles of combat that can be applied universally, there are four or five techniques worth exploring.

Funakoshi's early work depicted the T-stance, also known as '*renoji-dachi*' which, when the heels are lifted, becomes the fundamental posture of Te. From here the liberated, skipping type, footwork can be fully utilised which in some ways is reflective of the 'competition-styled' method of moving on the balls of the feet. Never static but paradoxically finding perpetual balance through being constantly unbalanced.

The basic '*kamae*' or 'guard position' of Te is also found in karate through the technique called '*morote-uke*', an augmented forearm block in which one fist is held at face height and the other floats by the elbow. This posture, is not too dissimilar, and perhaps even influenced by, the pose of early Queensbury Rules boxing posters of the nineteenth century. It allows for rapid strikes without chambering the fist to the hip or high under the armpit. *Morote-uke*, which in Te is called *meotode*, is the 'husband and wife' hands of Te mentioned by Funakoshi in *Karate-Dō Kyohan*. One hand supports the other and the two work in unison to form an effective offensive defence. Higa Kiyohiko has suggested that this form is likely to have evolved from use of the *koyumi* or 'short bow' which was once a fundamental weapon of Ryukyu Bujutsu and one Anko Asato was well versed in.

It's also worth considering that, despite the very diverse range of techniques studied in karate, competitive sparring favours just a few. The front jab, reverse punch and kicks delivered from the front leg. Experience reveals these to be the most efficient and effective in live combat and they are the basis upon which the rudimentary style of boxing called '*kashin-ti*' or 'battle hands' is taught in Te.

Another consideration is that the foremost fist taught in Funakoshi's time was '*ippon-ken*' the single point fist. This was Asato's favourite technique and has been shown to be directly related to the way in which weapons in Te are held. The single point fist, whether the point be a protruding index knuckle or thumb tip, enables for the striking of pressure-points. Such pressure-points were clearly known by Funakoshi but are rarely practised in dojo's today. Take the time to learn the locations of *tsubo*, and their dual role in both healing and fighting, and you will significantly enrich both your martial art skill and health.

The principles of Te are also simple and few in number. Avoid and enter simultaneously with no pause in between, rather than the 'block' then 'strike' preference of karate.

Another principle is the use of the forty-five degree angle as a line of entry. The key difference between the modern versions of karate kata and those of Okinawan tradition is generally the removal of this forty-five degree entry line. When you apply this with the principle of non-confrontation, 'avoid and enter', then you begin to practise *numba*, the way of maximising the effect of your own defence by working with the opponent's advance. That is, you advance forward into the attack but at a diagonal angle that heightens the effectiveness of your own strike using the momentum of the opponent's advance against them self. Additionally there are no retreating or 'back stepping' techniques in Te.

If the only way to learn Te technique is to feel it then nowhere else was that notion more true than in the presence of my *sempai* Isyado at the Bugeikan. He was relentless in ensuring I never moved on to another technique until the one I was on could be performed with competence under pressure.

This is the best way to learn martial arts. Direct, one to one and in small groups. The large organisations and governing bodies of the twentieth century have already served their initial purpose of spreading the popularity of styles around the world. But outside of organising competitions or providing block insurance policies for their members they are ultimately void of any real purpose moving into the future. Barely a hundred years on from the first organisations and the world is ready once again to return to a more holistic way of learning and training.

Karate-ka today can gain a foundation in a solid style and then begin to look outside for a teacher that appeals to them on a personal level. There is nothing wrong in this. No shame. In days past this was the way karate was learnt on Okinawa. No real 'schools' but teachers overseeing small groups, working together and supporting each other in a nourishing way. You trained with one teacher and the regime was prescribed for you, personally. If your teacher felt you would benefit from learning the technique of another they would likely set up the introduction for you.

At the Bugeikan the training is always focussed upon health and wellbeing. The current trend of seeking '*bunkai*' and effective 'defence applications' from kata is a phenomena that can only go so far before it descends into training that is ultimately destructive for longterm health and wellbeing. The real secret is not to develop powerful shoulders and musculature but to go inside and find the internal movements that will nourish the body and soul from within.

Modern day karate classes must be careful about focusing too much on fighting at the cost of losing other factors more important for wellbeing. Certainly physical training is the first important step towards leading a fulfilling life, but only if it is the correct physical training in accordance with proper movement dynamics.

If you think about it, there is a certain structure that most traditional karate classes follow but that few teachers even realise why. When you look for this structure you are able to gauge for yourself whether a class offers a complete training or is potentially focusing on too narrow a field to be of real 'long term' benefit to you.

Typically a class begins with preparatory exercises to free the body of stiffness, followed by basic training such as kata to coordinate the breath with movement. Partner training follows to encourage trainees to instinctively react to attacks without logical thought.

At the Bugeikan, Higa sensei will usually lead from this into kobudo and Te because training with weapons further helps to bring out the higher aspects of martial training such as 'extended awareness' before ending with meditation.

If the trainee is still stiff and struggles to enter a clear mindset then the remaining tension in the body can be released through the application of pressure to specific *tsubo's* to clear the 'blockage' such as shiatsu technique.

In essence, a well structured class along these lines is the path from action to in-action. A means by which your training can help to dissolve the daily accumulation of stress and fatigue that accumulates in the mind and body and which, if left unchecked, leads to poor health. Training in this way will liberate your mind to enter a peaceful, meditative state, a state of mind with 'no fixed ideas', known as *Munenmuso*.

Before a typical training session the mind and body are usually tense from the days earlier activities and through preparatory exercises you begin to release stress and begin to induce a relaxed mental state. The more relaxed the body and mind become the more active the workout can be without damaging the body or long term health.

Preparatory exercises help to warm-up, loosen, elongate and tone the soft tissues of the body. Such exercises should be performed in coordination with the breath, inhaling through the nose and exhaling through the mouth when stretching out or expanding, as when kicking or punching.

In this way the whole body, especially the joints, become flexible and allow for trainees to apply locks and techniques without the annoyance of aches and pains the following day. In the West, or any culture where lifestyles are more sedentary, extra emphasis should be placed on exercising the knees, hips and spine.

The next stage is to direct strength out from the hips and abdomen to develop the *hara* and enhance martial technique. It's important to learn how to breathe deeply by drawing air into the lungs using the lower abdominal muscles and how to exhale appropriately to support technique.

Most martial art techniques begin in the feet and are directed by the waist to the hands; in the same manner young children move. In this way, with a body free of tension and working with the breath, your intrinsic energy will rise up and flow freely to be directed by the mind upon a single focussed point.

After a training session along these lines a trainee is well prepared for seated meditation. Moving from action to inaction the 'flow' of a traditional martial arts workout is designed to noticeably change your brainwave patterns from its usual active 'beta' state to a more sedate, yet aware 'alpha' or even 'theta' pattern.

When teachers of karate and kobudo understand and use this structure in their classes they at once move beyond the fear-motivated focus of "combat efficiency" that has plagued the majority of western dojos of late and instead begin to truly help students nourish their health and enrich their lives.

Be mindful though. Master Itosu once warned:

'Do not overexert yourself during practise otherwise the ki will rise up, your face and eyes will turn red and your body will be harmed.'

A final important aspect concerning the development of martial arts is your personal practice. My training over the years has taken me away from mainstream classes to the extent of usually training one to one with a select number of skilled sensei, or alone in the solitude of nature. It is a rare path and one that's not for everyone. However the important thing for all karate-ka is to develop your own personal practice.

Few are committed enough or even able to train daily in a class environment, but that is ok. The trick is to ensure you do a little every day. Funakoshi would train for short periods of say ten to fifteen minutes several times a day. His main training periods were during the late night or early morning. It is not necessary to train for an hour or two every day. Often it is not practical either.

Asato's house was said to be like a dojo, with training devices in several rooms so that he could rehearse and hone techniques as he moved about his home.

"Find ways to bring your karate into your daily life."

Exercise upon waking, if only for five minutes, rehearse kata during a break, stretch the arms above the head and breathe. Karate is a life art.

The whole time you see your karate training as something 'extra' in your day then you will find reasons why sometimes you cannot 'fit' it into your day. Discipline leads to good health so train daily, even if only for short periods. This is the approach of Te and karate as a life art for internal self development.

For me, ultimately, this journey has been an enlightening and deeply enriching process. It's not over yet and I have a long way to go. Coming full circle I now realise that the 'old way' of karate is often not what most people think. Yes its techniques are more effective for self-defence than it's sporting cousin but this is achieved through softness not hardness. The real essence is health. When you look and find the true 'old school' masters you'll find their movements are not hard, stiff and robust but soft, flowing and fast. Today Goju-ryu karate is notoriously considered a 'hard' style but if you search deep enough you will find those skilled in the old way of moving which is very different, more fluid and far more like Chinese kung-fu.

The techniques of Tomari-te, little known today but studied by Higa sensei's grandfather under the Kosaku Matsumora line, is also soft and fluid in nature. It's roots are found in China and stem from the internal kung-fu style called Hsing-yi. When Tomari-te blended with Shuri-te the five core striking methods of Hsing-yi likely became the five fundamental '*uke*' techniques of modern karate, and the back-stance brought a new movement dynamic to the art too. The early origins of this style are found in Chinese spear-fighting.

Shuri-te was a style mostly influenced by Te proper. It's early movements were also fluid and yielding supported on a unique footwork and upright posture. Techniques and strategies of Te were handed down from the noble warrior clans of Shuri and blended with ideas of the time from Tomari and the military arts of China through visiting envoys. Certain techniques, as already mentioned, came directly from weaponry training and is the reason for the light and nimble footwork.

As weapons became less common on the island the footwork started to become more rooted. Eventually Shuri-te and Tomari-te blended to become the basis of a collection of styles called Shorin, from which Shotokan derives. About the same time, the methods of Naha-te became known as Shorei.

Everything changes with time. About two hundred years ago the way of walking for mainland Japanese was totally different than today. Back then, depending on your class status, you walked differently. Peasant farmers were often hunched with a movement that exaggerated bow-shaped legs. Merchants walked with head lowered and hands upon the front of the thighs, often bowing and kowtowing to customers. While the Samurai held their head high with shoulders back and swaggered in a peculiar way. In feudal Japan it was possible to guess someone's class by not only observing their costume but the way they walked and moved too. It was only with the abolition of that defunct social structure that people started to walk in the more westernised manner seen today. Similar comparisons can be made in Okinawa.

If you want to explore the 'old' then examine the movement dynamics of the culture karate came from. I have found that the dynamics of Te are more reflective of ancient Japanese *bujutsu* which was more fluid and circular in nature when compared with *bujutsu* styles from the 17th century onwards.

The build of the karate-ka today is also not the same as that of yesteryear. Neither is their longevity. In his last recorded interview Uehara Seikichi, who lived and taught to a hundred, reflected:

> *'It bothers me that recently many masters of karate die young. This is very different from the past. I believe there are errors in their training, it does not permit them to remain physically healthy. their daily training tenses the body and legs and consequently they develop arthritis and other problems. In the old days training was different. We used to stretch our backs, raise our shoulders, stretch up with our arms and then downwards expelling the air. natural breathing is very important for correctly training in bujutsu.'*

This is how my training has evolved. Yes the combative aspects are there, based as they are upon real life experiences, but ultimately the emphasis is on health and the preservation of life. Because without health nothing else matters.

As for my search for the old to understand the new?

The old, the new. This is a matter of time.
In all things you must have a clear mind.

**Continue your journey at
www.thekarateka.com**

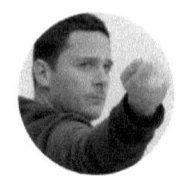

Joel Reeves has been training in karate for over thirty years. His unique approach has taken him out of the mainstream dojo in search of some of the most noted teachers of Okinawan bujutsu.

Presently living in England he teaches Okinawan martial arts and works as a professional Shiatsu Therapist specialising in the treatment of injuries, back pain and stress related illness.

To contact the author visit:
www.thekarateka.com

Lightning Source UK Ltd.
Milton Keynes UK
UKHW01f1748060818
326846UK00001B/380/P